Intermittent
FASTING

FOR WOMEN OVER

50

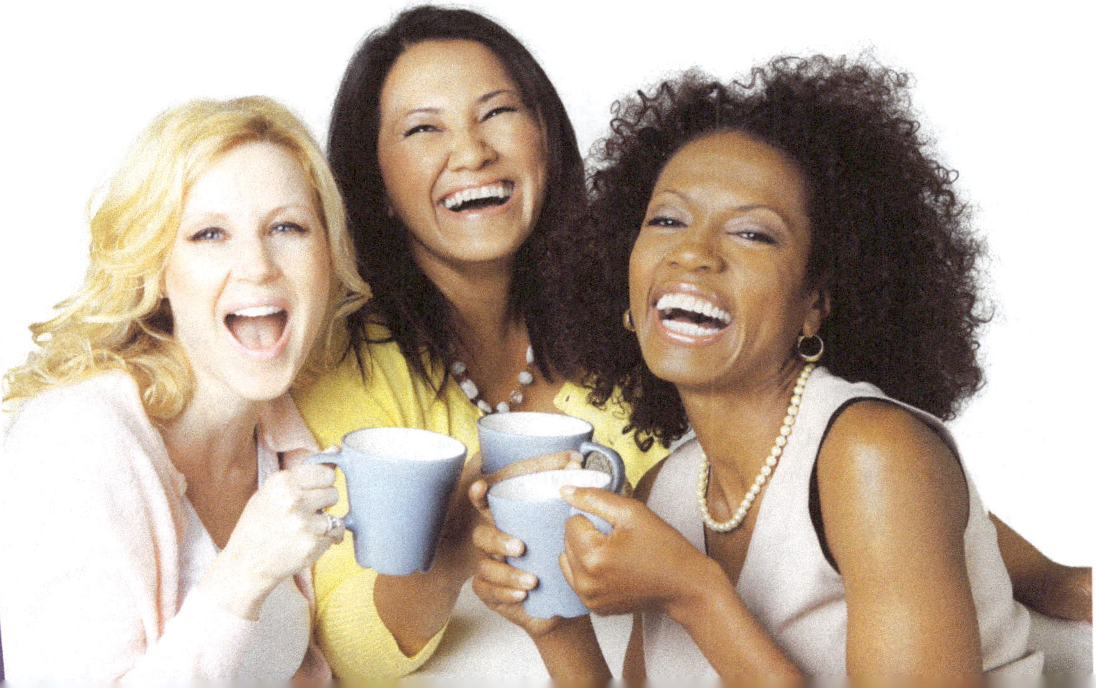

INTRODUCTION

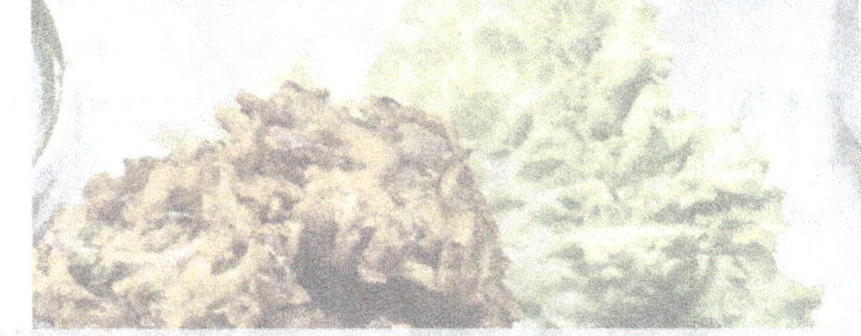

Welcome to the golden chapter of your life, where the wisdom of experience meets the excitement of new beginnings. It's a time when self-care isn't just a luxury; it's essential. What better way to honor your journey than by embracing the transformative practice of intermittent fasting? This isn't just a book; it's a warm and welcoming conversation between friends, a collection of whispers of wisdom shared over garden fences, and the empowering cheers of a community that knows the strength of women like us.

Imagine sitting down with a cup of your favorite tea, leafing through pages that feel like letters from a dear friend. That's the essence of "Intermittent Fasting for Women Over 50." This guide is as warm as a comforting hug, as friendly as a heartwarming chat, as factual as a trusted companion, and as encouraging as the morning sun.

We'll start by opening the door to understanding what intermittent fasting is all about – it's not a passing trend but a timeless approach to eating that can seamlessly blend into your lifestyle, just like your favorite pair of comfortable yet flattering jeans. We'll dispel any myths, shed light on the science, and most importantly, celebrate the unique benefits of being fabulous over 50s who are aging and genuinely ageless.

Preparation is a vital foundation for our intermittent fasting journey, like meticulously planning the perfect soirée. Just as you ensure every detail is in place for a memorable gathering, we'll ensure that every aspect of your health and well-being is considered as we embark on this transformative path.

Getting the green light from your healthcare providers is our foremost priority. We'll explore the importance of open communication with your medical team, discussing any concerns or questions you might have and ensuring that intermittent fasting aligns with your unique health needs. It's like having a trusted advisor guiding you on this empowering journey.

But preparation goes beyond just the physical. We'll also delve into the mental and emotional aspects, helping you prepare your mind for the changes ahead. Like setting the stage for a heartfelt conversation with a dear friend, we'll address any doubts, fears, or anxieties, allowing you to approach intermittent fasting with confidence and self-assuredness.

Creating an environment as nurturing as the bond you share with your closest friends is essential. Just as your social circle provides support and encouragement, we'll help you establish a support network for your fasting journey. This might involve sharing your goals with loved ones, joining a community of like-minded women, or finding an accountability partner who will be there to cheer you on.

We aim to ensure that the soil is fertile and enriched with positivity and resilience before you plant the seeds of your new, healthy habits. This preparation phase is the cornerstone of your success in embracing intermittent fasting as a natural and sustainable part of your vibrant life.

Nutrition is not overlooked. We'll delve into the art of choosing nutrient-dense foods that don't merely fill us but nourish us deeply. We'll learn to keep our hydration as vibrant as a blooming flower and explore how supplements can play a role in our symphony of health. This chapter is the spice rack of our fasting journey – brimming with variety and zest.

And what's a good book without addressing the real-life plot twists? We'll tackle common side effects and learn how to gracefully navigate them. Life is full of surprises, so we'll equip ourselves with strategies to adapt our fasting schedule to the ever-changing rhythms of life. Additionally, we'll understand when and why it might be time to break a fast, attuning ourselves to the wisdom of our bodies.

UNDERSTANDING INTERMITTENT FASTING

Welcome, my fabulous fellow over-50s! If you've been hearing the buzz about intermittent fasting and are curious to see what it's all about, you're in the right place. This isn't just another diet fad; it's a lifestyle sweeping through our age group, and for good reason. Let's cozy up with a cup of tea and chat about this journey that might be the game-changer we've been looking for. We'll explore what intermittent fasting means, peel back the layers of science to understand how it works, discover its benefits, especially for us, and debunk some of those pesky myths. Ready to dive in? Let's turn the page and start our adventure into intermittent fasting.

Defining Intermittent Fasting

Intermittent fasting is a versatile and empowering approach to nourishing our bodies, much like orchestrating a symphony of eating habits. Imagine your day as a composition, and intermittent fasting is the conductor, guiding when the music of consumption begins and when it takes its intermission. It's not a rigid dietary regimen telling you what specific dishes to savor; instead, it's about the elegant choreography of time.

One popular method is the 16/8 approach, where you enjoy your meals within an 8-hour window and abstain from eating for the remaining 16 hours. It's like setting the rhythm of your day to a harmonious tune, aligning your eating schedule with your lifestyle. Others might resonate with the 5:2 pattern, allowing them to eat normally five days a week while taking a unique pause on two non-consecutive days, limiting their calorie intake to around 500-600 calories. This method offers flexibility and balance, like a well-composed melody with pauses and crescendos. Another intriguing option is the 'Eat-Stop-Eat' method. Here, you choose one or two days a week to abstain from food for 24 hours. It's akin to a brief sabbatical for your digestive system, allowing it to reset and rejuvenate. Whichever method you choose, intermittent fasting allows you to press the pause button on eating, providing your body with a well-deserved vacation from the continuous task of digestion. It's a symphony of control, allowing you to harmonize your health, metabolism, and well-being with the rhythms of your own life.

The Science Behind Intermittent Fasting

Indeed, here's an expanded explanation of the science behind intermittent fasting in a clear and approachable manner, following the example in the original text:

Picture your body as a finely tuned engine. Ordinarily, it relies on glucose, the energy it extracts from the food you eat. When you take a pause from eating, your body's glucose reservoir eventually runs low, prompting it to search for an alternate energy source. Here's where the star of the show enters – your body's fat stores. It initiates a fascinating process called ketosis, where those stored fats are transformed into energy. It's like a captivating shift in the plot, with Fat stepping into the lead role.

But the magic of intermittent fasting isn't limited to fat utilization; it's a multi-act performance of health benefits. Fasting has the potential to reduce inflammation, giving your body a well-deserved break from the aches and discomfort that can arise. It's akin to a calming interlude in the story, offering relief and soothing relief to the audience.

Intermittent fasting also has a pivotal role in enhancing insulin sensitivity. Think of it as a conductor fine-tuning the orchestra for perfect harmony in your metabolic symphony. Your body becomes more adept at efficiently managing insulin, a vital hormone in your body's operation.

UNDERSTANDING INTERMITTENT FASTING

A remarkable facet of intermittent fasting is providing respite to your diligent digestive system. Just as actors take a break between acts, fasting allows your digestive organs to recharge and refresh. It's a moment of relaxation in the ongoing narrative of digestion.

And now, the grand finale – scientific research suggests that intermittent fasting can trigger essential cellular repair processes, including autophagy. Imagine autophagy as your cells engaging in a deep cleaning session. They tidy up, eliminate debris, and recycle damaged components to construct new, healthy ones. It's like the behind-the-scenes crew preparing the stage for the next act.

Intermittent fasting isn't solely about weight management; it's a symphony of metabolic transformations, offering a range of benefits that extend far beyond the scale. It's a journey where your body undergoes a profound metamorphosis, repairs itself, and rejuvenates. At the same time, you take the role of the conductor, orchestrating your own health and well-being.

Benefits Specific to Women Over 50

Now, why is this particularly fab for those of us women over the hill? As we get a little older, our metabolism isn't what it used to be. Intermittent fasting can kick it up a notch. Remember those hormonal rollercoasters? Well, fasting can help level out those bumps by stabilizing insulin levels, which can have a domino effect on other hormones, like estrogen and progesterone. Plus, it can be a great way to manage weight, which is often more stubborn than ever in our 50s. It can improve brain health, too, keeping our wits as sharp as our fashion sense. And heart health? Intermittent fasting can improve blood pressure and cholesterol levels, keeping that ticker happy and robust.

Common Myths and Misconceptions

Myth #1: Fasting Slows Down Your Metabolism

The truth is that well-executed intermittent fasting can actually boost your metabolism. By allowing your body to tap into fat stores for energy during fasting periods, you can encourage healthy weight management and metabolic efficiency. It's more like giving your metabolism a chance to adapt and work more effectively.

Myth #2: You Can't Exercise While Fasting

Contrary to this belief, exercising during fasting is not only safe but can be highly beneficial. Many women find that combining intermittent fasting with exercise helps them achieve their fitness goals and improve their overall well-being. It's like giving your workouts an edge, promoting fat loss and muscle preservation.

Myth #3: Fasting Causes Muscle Loss

Intermittent fasting, when done correctly, doesn't inherently lead to muscle loss. In fact, it can help preserve lean muscle mass while your body utilizes fat stores for energy. Think of it as a way to maintain your body's strength and tone while shedding excess fat.

UNDERSTANDING INTERMITTENT FASTING

Myth #4: Skipping Breakfast Is Unhealthy
While breakfast is often touted as the most important meal of the day, intermittent fasting isn't about skipping breakfast for the sake of it. It's about aligning your eating schedule with your body's natural rhythms and needs. For some women, starting their eating window later in the day feels more natural and energizing.

Myth #5: You Must Follow a Specific Fasting Schedule
Intermittent fasting isn't a one-size-fits-all approach. It's highly adaptable to your preferences and lifestyle. You can tailor your fasting window to suit your daily routine and comfort, whether it's the 16/8 method, the 5:2 pattern, or any other variation that aligns with your needs and goals.
In the world of intermittent fasting, dispelling these myths is crucial. It's about understanding the science behind it, listening to your body's cues, and finding the approach that suits you best. Remember, it's a flexible and empowering journey, and your health and well-being always come first.
Alright, my friends, we've just scratched the surface of intermittent fasting, but what a ride, huh? It's clear that this isn't just a trend; it's a way of eating that could make a big difference in how we feel and live. Remember, this journey is personal. What works for one person might not work for another, so it's all about finding your groove and listening to your body. As we move on to the next chapter, keep your mind open and consider how this could fit into your life. Could intermittent fasting be your ticket to feeling fabulous in your 50s and beyond? Let's find out together!

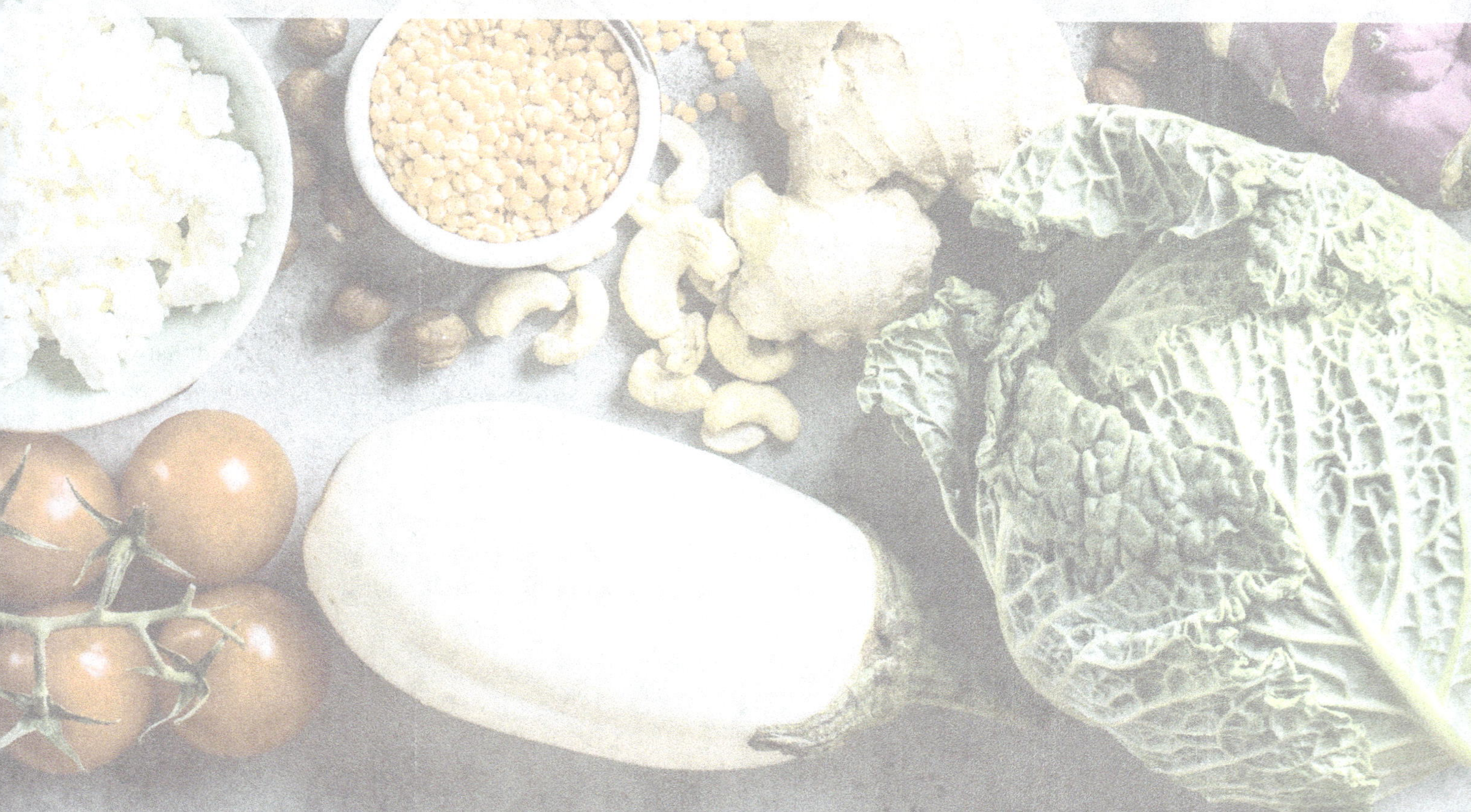

PREPARING FOR INTERMITTENT FASTING

Just like when you're prepping for that garden party, you need to think about who's coming, what they like, what the theme is—every little detail matters. It's the same with intermittent fasting. You'll want to personalize this plan to fit you like your favorite pair of comfy yet oh-so-chic jeans. We're not just throwing things together and hoping it works out; we're thoughtfully selecting every piece, from the timing of our meals to the snacks we'll have on hand for breaking our fast.

We'll also talk about aligning our fasting schedule with our body's natural rhythms, like planning the party when the garden is in full bloom. This way, we're working with our bodies, not against them. Think about those times when you're naturally not hungry and how you might use those to your advantage.

And remember the social aspect! We would only plan a party if we considered our guests and the same goes for our fasting plan. We'll think about how to handle social situations, like brunch with the girls or family dinners, to achieve our goals. It's about being prepared with a little spiel on why you're not eating the birthday cake at 3 p.m. because, guess what, your eating window opens at 5 p.m., and you're sticking to it.

Think of this chapter as the ultimate party planning checklist for your intermittent fasting journey. By the end, you'll have your RSVPs from your healthcare team, your goals will be set like a date in the diary, and your environment will be as ready as your garden decked out in fairy lights. You're not just going with the flow; you're creating the flow that will carry you to a healthier, happier you. So, let's turn that music up, get our planning hats on, and get ready to throw the best intermittent fasting party for our health!

Consulting with Healthcare Providers

Imagine you're planning a trip to a destination you've never been to before. You'd likely consult a travel agent. That's what your healthcare provider is regarding intermittent fasting—a guide to uncharted territory. They can run a quick 'itinerary' check on your health to ensure fasting is a good fit for you. This might include a chat about your medical history, current medications, and health concerns like blood sugar levels or blood pressure. It's not just about getting a nod of approval but also about tailoring the fasting experience to your body's unique needs. Maybe you have a thyroid issue or diabetes, and your fasting plan needs to accommodate that. Your provider might suggest monitoring your nutrient levels or adjusting medications. It's like getting a custom weather report for your health to ensure you pack the right gear for the journey ahead.

Mental Preparation and Setting Realistic Goals

Now, on to prepping our minds. Imagine you're going to grow a garden. You wouldn't just throw seeds on the soil and hope for the best. You'd plan, prepare the soil, and choose the right seeds—the same goes for fasting. Begin with manageable goals. If a 16-hour fast seems too much, why not try 12 hours? After all, much of that time, you might be asleep! Celebrate the small wins, like choosing a healthy snack to break your fast or simply completing a fasting period without giving in to temptation. And on those days when things don't go as planned? Don't beat yourself up. Be as compassionate with yourself as you would be with your best friend. Adapt and keep moving forward. This is a lifestyle change, not a quick fix, so give yourself the grace to grow into it.

PREPARING FOR INTERMITTENT FASTING

Creating a Supportive Environment

Just as you wouldn't plant a sun-loving flower in the shade, it's essential to create an environment that nurtures your fasting goals. Starting with your kitchen, make it a place that syncs seamlessly with your fasting lifestyle. Consider bidding farewell to that tempting cookie jar on the counter and embracing a beautiful bowl of fresh fruit for your eating window. Your kitchen can be your ally, motivating you to make healthier choices effortlessly.

When it comes to family and friends, open and honest communication is vital. Have a heart-to-heart conversation with your loved ones about your fasting goals. Perhaps your partner is eager to embark on this journey with you, or your friends are willing to adjust their brunch plans to accommodate your fasting schedule. Remember, socializing can sometimes revolve around something other than food. Suggests activities like leisure walks, a cozy movie night, or a fun craft evening. These alternatives allow you to maintain those valuable social connections while staying true to your fasting routine.

A supportive environment is the fertile soil where your fasting journey can take root. It's your anchor, empowering you to not only follow your fasting plan but also integrate it seamlessly into your lifestyle. This isn't just a diet; it's a sustainable way of living that aligns with your health and well-being.

Alright, beautiful ladies, we're armed with a doctor's advice, goals that make us giddy, and a home that will support us like the best of friends. Preparing for intermittent fasting isn't just about the physical stuff; it's about gearing up emotionally and mentally, too. Remember to be kind to yourself through this process. It's not about perfection; it's about making a positive change. With a solid plan, we're ready to embark on this fasting journey with confidence and a support system that's as strong and fabulous as we are. Let's raise a glass (of water for now!) to us – we will rock this!

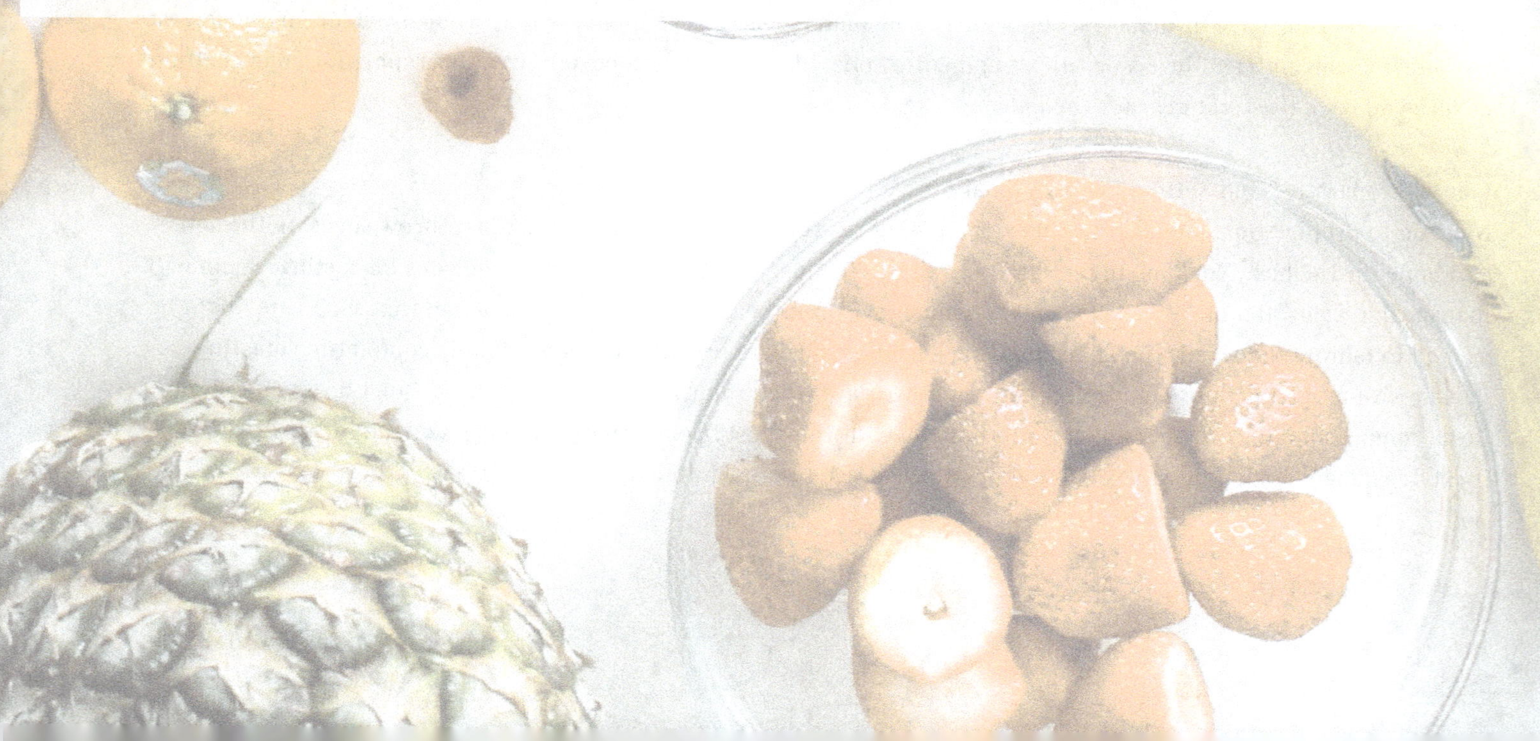

INTERMITTENT FASTING AND NUTRITION

Imagine your eating window as the VIP section of a concert – only the best should get a pass. This is the time to be intentional about your consumption, making each bite count. Think fiber-rich veggies, lean proteins, whole grains, and those fats that make your heart and brain thank you, like avocados and nuts. These are the nutritional rock stars that'll keep you feeling full and satisfied, which is especially important when you're on a fasting schedule.

And when it comes to hydration, think of water as the headliner of your personal health festival. It's about keeping the rhythm throughout the day, not just guzzling water during your eating hours but also during fasting. Plus, staying hydrated keeps the dreaded hunger pangs at bay, often mistaken for thirst cues.

Lastly, let's fine-tune our understanding of supplements like a sound check before the show. We'll consider if there's a need for an encore as a vitamin or mineral supplement, especially when our eating might not hit all the high notes of our nutritional needs. Remember, supplements should complement, not replace, a symphony of healthy foods.

With our plates and glasses set to the tune of health and vitality, we'll be eating to the rhythm of well-being, and that's a concert worth attending every day. Now, with a better understanding of how to orchestrate our nutrition, we're ready to waltz gracefully into the practicalities of making intermittent fasting a harmonious part of our lifestyle.

Nutrient-Dense Foods for Optimal Health

Imagine walking into a vibrant artist's studio, where your palette is filled with the rich colors of nutrient-packed foods. Your canvas? It's your plate, waiting for you to create nourishing and delicious meals. Start with a bed of lush leafy greens—think spinach, kale, and Swiss chard. These leaves are more than just a pretty backdrop; they're packed with vitamins, iron, and calcium, supporting your health in more ways than one. Now, add a beautiful slice of salmon, glistening with heart-healthy omega-3 fatty acids. These nutrients are essential for brain health and keeping your joints moving gracefully. And don't forget to include a handful of berries—blueberries, raspberries, strawberries. These little gems contain fiber, vitamins, and antioxidants that combat those pesky free radicals. This is not just a meal; it's the fuel that keeps your body running smoothly, reviving your energy and making you feel ready to conquer your day.

Hydration and Electrolyte Balance

Maintaining proper hydration is as crucial as nurturing a lush garden. Just as plants wither without adequate water, our bodies simply can't function optimally. While you've likely heard the guideline of drinking eight glasses of water a day, it's essential to recognize that during fasting, your body may require a little extra attention in the hydration department.

Hydration isn't just about plain water; crafting a hydrating experience that resonates with your body's needs. Add a pinch of mineral-rich salt, a dash of magnesium powder, or a slice of potassium-packed cucumber to your water. These elements can work together to create a revitalizing elixir, not only quenching your thirst but also replenishing vital electrolytes. Picture this elixir as a conductor, orchestrating the harmonious functioning of your cells, keeping them vibrant and full of vitality.

INTERMITTENT FASTING AND NUTRITION

Remember to explore the world of herbal teas. Sipping on these flavorful infusions not only contributes to your hydration goals but also brings a unique set of benefits. Different herbal teas can soothe digestion, calm the mind, or invigorate your senses, all while keeping your body hydrated. They're like a symphony of flavors and wellness in a single cup.

Just as you keep your favorite sunglasses indispensable and ready for use, make a habit of keeping a bottle of water within arm's reach. It becomes an ever-present companion, a refreshing source of vitality, ensuring you're always equipped to provide your body with the hydration it craves. Hydration is the foundation of your well-being, and it's within your power to keep it in perfect harmony.

Supplements and Intermittent Fasting

Lastly, let's explore the world of supplements. Think of them as the reliable safety net for your nutrition, ready to catch you if your diet misses the mark. Before you consider adding a multivitamin or fish oil to your daily routine, consult with a nutritionist to understand where your meals might need to be improved. Are your bones craving more calcium? Does your body need an extra Vitamin D? Supplements are like supporting acts, stepping up when your diet isn't providing all the necessary nutrients. Remember, they're supplements, not the main attraction. Prioritize obtaining your vitamins and minerals from whole foods, which your body can absorb more effectively. Consider supplements as the encore to an already impressive performance. Your health and well-being take center stage.

Alright, my lovelies, as we close this chapter, remember that what we put on our plates is just as important as the timing of our meals. We want to nourish our bodies with all the good stuff – think of it like high-quality fuel for a luxury car, which, let's face it, we all are. Keeping hydrated is like giving that car the right oil, and supplements can be the polish that keeps it shiny. Intermittent fasting isn't just about losing weight or ticking health goals; it's a way to show love to our bodies by choosing the best and ensuring we're as nourished and hydrated as a well-kept garden. In the next chapter, we'll dig into how to handle the bumps on the road and keep cruising smoothly on our intermittent fasting journey!

MANAGING CHALLENGES AND SIDE EFFECTS

My dear circle of fasting friends, let's gather around the table (even if it's metaphorically for now) and have an honest chat, the kind we'd have over a leisurely cup of coffee. When we step into the world of intermittent fasting, we're embarking on an exciting but sometimes challenging adventure. It's like setting out on a road trip; we expect smooth highways, but we also prepare for the occasional pothole. So, as we venture into this chapter, we'll map out the potential roadblocks and learn the savvy ways to maneuver around them.

We'll explore the common side effects as though we're sharing remedies at a book club meeting—sharing those tried-and-true tips for easing headaches or managing that mid-afternoon slump. This chapter will be our little toolbox, filled with all the practical gadgets to fix the minor hiccups along the way. And just like you might adjust a recipe to your taste, we'll talk about tailoring your fasting schedule. Hence, it fits into your life as seamlessly as your favorite sweater on a chilly evening.

And then, there's the art of knowing when to take a step back, when to indulge in self-care, and perhaps break your fast because your body is asking for it. It's not about waving a white flag; it's about honoring your health and well-being above all else. We'll learn to listen to our bodies with the attentiveness of a devoted friend because that's what they are—our lifelong companions.

As we turn these pages, we'll learn how to sway with the rhythm of intermittent fasting, not missing a beat even when life throws us a curveball. We'll weave the wisdom of our bodies with the science of fasting, creating a tapestry that tells the story of wellness, resilience, and balance. So, let's step forward confidently, knowing that we have the strategies, the understanding, and the heart to navigate this path with poise and grace. Ready to tackle these challenges head-on? Let's turn the page and begin.

Navigating Common Side Effects and Their Solutions

Stepping into intermittent fasting can feel like learning a new dance routine. Just like the initial awkward steps, you might encounter some side effects. Perhaps you've experienced that pesky, headachy feeling that sneaks up on you like an unwelcome party guest. Or the occasional grumpiness that makes you feel like you're turning into a bear without its winter hibernation. These are familiar tunes your body might play as it adjusts to the fasting rhythm.

To ease these challenges, hydration becomes your trusty companion—it's the background music that keeps everything harmonious. A pinch of salt in your water isn't just a flavor enhancer; it's a quick remedy for those nagging headaches that can sometimes accompany fasting. If your energy is dipping and you need a pick-me-up, reach for a comforting black coffee or a refreshing cup of green tea. These beverages are like a solo performance in your daily symphony—stimulating without breaking your fast. Don't forget the power of movement, too. A gentle stretch or a stroll around the block can work wonders to shake off the fasting funk, just like a refreshing interlude in your day.

For those moments when you need a bit of extra care, it's okay to pamper yourself. Remember, this is a lifestyle shift, and it deserves the same patience and nurturing you'd provide to a young sapling growing into a sturdy tree.

MANAGING CHALLENGES AND SIDE EFFECTS

My dear circle of fasting friends, let's gather around the table (even if it's metaphorically for now) and have an honest chat, the kind we'd have over a leisurely cup of coffee. When we step into the world of intermittent fasting, we're embarking on an exciting but sometimes challenging adventure. It's like setting out on a road trip; we expect smooth highways, but we also prepare for the occasional pothole. So, as we venture into this chapter, we'll map out the potential roadblocks and learn the savvy ways to maneuver around them.

We'll explore the common side effects as though we're sharing remedies at a book club meeting—sharing those tried-and-true tips for easing headaches or managing that mid-afternoon slump. This chapter will be our little toolbox, filled with all the practical gadgets to fix the minor hiccups along the way. And just like you might adjust a recipe to your taste, we'll talk about tailoring your fasting schedule. Hence, it fits into your life as seamlessly as your favorite sweater on a chilly evening. And then, there's the art of knowing when to take a step back, when to indulge in self-care, and perhaps break your fast because your body is asking for it. It's not about waving a white flag; it's about honoring your health and well-being above all else. We'll learn to listen to our bodies with the attentiveness of a devoted friend because that's what they are—our lifelong companions.

As we turn these pages, we'll learn how to sway with the rhythm of intermittent fasting, not missing a beat even when life throws us a curveball. We'll weave the wisdom of our bodies with the science of fasting, creating a tapestry that tells the story of wellness, resilience, and balance. So, let's step forward confidently, knowing that we have the strategies, the understanding, and the heart to navigate this path with poise and grace. Ready to tackle these challenges head-on? Let's turn the page and begin.

Navigating Common Side Effects and Their Solutions

Stepping into intermittent fasting can feel like learning a new dance routine. Just like the initial awkward steps, you might encounter some side effects. Perhaps you've experienced that pesky, headachy feeling that sneaks up on you like an unwelcome party guest. Or the occasional grumpiness that makes you feel like you're turning into a bear without its winter hibernation. These are familiar tunes your body might play as it adjusts to the fasting rhythm.

To ease these challenges, hydration becomes your trusty companion—it's the background music that keeps everything harmonious. A pinch of salt in your water isn't just a flavor enhancer; it's a quick remedy for those nagging headaches that can sometimes accompany fasting. If your energy is dipping and you need a pick-me-up, reach for a comforting black coffee or a refreshing cup of green tea. These beverages are like a solo performance in your daily symphony—stimulating without breaking your fast. Don't forget the power of movement, too. A gentle stretch or a stroll around the block can work wonders to shake off the fasting funk, just like a refreshing interlude in your day.

For those moments when you need a bit of extra care, it's okay to pamper yourself. Remember, this is a lifestyle shift, and it deserves the same patience and nurturing you'd provide to a young sapling growing into a sturdy tree.

Adapting the Fasting Schedule to Your Life

Now, let's talk about the art of seamlessly weaving intermittent fasting into the fabric of your daily life. Just as you might tailor a dress to fit perfectly for a special occasion, your fasting schedule can be adjusted to align with your life's events. Do you have a grandkid's early soccer game to attend? Consider breaking your fast with a healthy snack on the sidelines. Or there's a dinner party that calls for a slight shift in your eating window. The beauty of intermittent fasting is that it's not rigid; it's designed to be as adaptable as your life requires.

MANAGING CHALLENGES AND SIDE EFFECTS

Think of your fasting schedule as your personal playlist—it should bring you joy and suit your unique vibe. There's no need to dance to someone else's beat. Like a seasoned improviser, you'll learn to adapt and embrace unexpected moments. A late meeting? No problem, just adjust your eating window. This isn't a one-size-fits-all approach; it's custom-tailored by you, for you.

When to Break the Fast Early

And what about those days when you simply aren't feeling your best? That's your cue to tune into your body's whispers before they become shouts. Feeling weak or dizzy is akin to the warning lights on your car's dashboard—signals that should not be ignored. In such cases, it's perfectly acceptable to break your fast early. So, what should you reach for? Choose something wholesome and gentle on an empty stomach, like a small handful of almonds, a ripe banana, or a nourishing smoothie. This helps you ease back into eating comfortably.

Your body is the show's star, and if it's not ready to perform, your priority is to take care of it rather than pushing through the last act. There's strength in recognizing when to take a step back, to nourish and rest. Intermittent fasting is a journey, not a destination, and sometimes journeys need unexpected pit stops. Remember, each day is a new scene, and you're the director—feel free to adjust the script as needed. There's grace in flexibility and wisdom in listening to your body. Tomorrow is a fresh start, another chance to embrace fasting and continue writing your unique health story.

So, my lovely ladies, as we wrap up this chapter, remember that intermittent fasting isn't about toughing it out through the hard times. It's about tuning in to your body's needs and finding your unique fasting flow. Side effects might come and go, just like fashion trends, but knowing how to manage them keeps you feeling timeless and fabulous. Adapting the fasting schedule to your lifestyle ensures this isn't just a fad—it's a sustainable part of your life. And knowing when to break your fast early—that's wisdom. This kind only comes with experience and listening to the deep, intuitive knowledge of your own body. With grace and flexibility, we'll continue to navigate this fasting path, making it work for us in the most nourishing way possible. Now, let's turn the page and continue this journey with confidence and self-compassion.

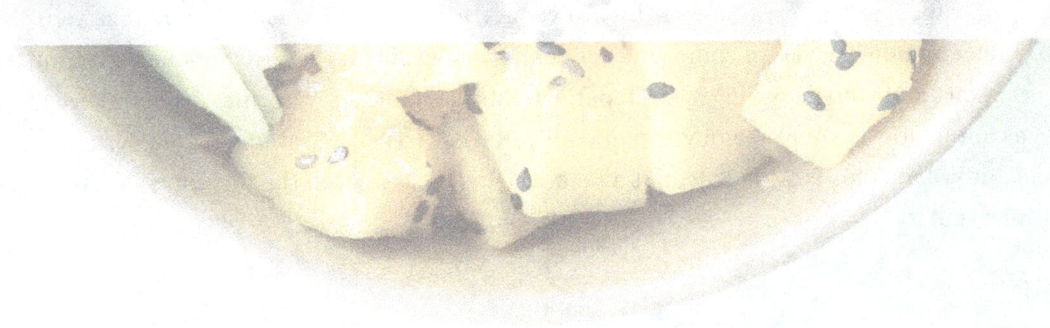

ADVANCED STRATEGIES AND LONGEVITY

Think of this chapter as the spice cabinet of your intermittent fasting journey. Just like the right herbs and spices can turn a simple meal into a gourmet feast, the strategies we're about to unpack can transform your fasting experience from basic to brilliant. We're not just skimming the surface; we're going full gourmet chef with our fasting routine, adding layers of flavor with exercise, ensuring the taste remains exquisite with long-term habits, and infusing everything with the anti-aging essence of autophagy.

Imagine entering the part of the garden where the more exotic plants bloom. Such a bloom promises longevity and vitality. That's the essence of this chapter. It's about understanding the synergy between fasting, movement, and cellular health. This is where you take control, steering your fasting practice into uncharted territories of wellness and vitality. So, tie up those laces for the exercise of life, fine-tune your daily habits for a symphony of health, and prepare to embrace the science that keeps you not just going but thriving as we unlock the secrets to a well-loved life. Now, let's deepen our understanding and commitment as we move into the heart of advanced intermittent fasting.

Combining Intermittent Fasting with Exercise

When you lace up those sneakers or unfurl that yoga mat while fasting, you're setting the stage for some severe fat-burning drama. Your body, having used up its quick-access energy reserves, is now ready to turn to fat storage for a standing ovation. It's like having a VIP pass to your stored fat, and exercise is the bouncer letting you through the velvet rope. It's not about going hardcore or busting out grueling workouts unless that's your jam. It's about being consistent and finding joy in movement. It could be a dance class that makes you feel alive, a strength training session that leaves you feeling powerful, or a pilates routine that centers you. The point is, when exercise meets fasting, it's less about the calories burned and more about the empowerment gained. You're forging a partnership with your body, understanding its cues, and reaping the full benefits of your fasted state.

Long-Term Maintenance

The trick to making intermittent fasting a long-term gig is like perfecting your grandmother's signature dish—it takes a little tweaking, a dash of patience, and a sprinkle of love. It's about finding your 'sweet spot'—that balance between your fasting protocol and the rest of your life. Introduce new, healthy foods that tantalize your taste buds. Keep a journal to reflect on how far you've come, and set gentle, achievable targets. Remember, intermittent fasting is not just a series of start and stop days; it's a woven pattern into the fabric of your life. It's about creating a tapestry of habits as automatic as your morning cup of coffee. Revisit your motivations regularly, adjust as you go, and if you hit a snag, it's okay. This is a lifestyle, not a race, and every step, even the tiny ones, is a part of your journey to a healthier you.

ADVANCED STRATEGIES AND LONGEVITY

Autophagy and Anti-Aging Benefits

Our bodies are intricate, self-sustaining ecosystems, tirelessly working to maintain balance and health. Within this marvel of biology lies a remarkable process known as autophagy – a term derived from the Greek words "auto," meaning self, and "phagy," meaning eating. Think of it as the silent janitor of your body, dutifully performing its tasks. At the same time, you slumber or deep into your fasting period. Autophagy is the biological equivalent of hitting the reset button, providing your cells with an opportunity to tidy up, discard accumulated waste, and emerge more robust and vibrant. In the following discussion, we'll delve into the fascinating world of autophagy, exploring how this cellular clean-up process contributes to your overall well-being and why it's gained recognition as a potential anti-aging mechanism.

Imagine your cells as miniature factories, constantly producing and degrading cellular components to maintain function and health. Over time, these cellular factories accumulate waste and damaged materials. This buildup is where autophagy comes into play. It's a meticulously regulated process where your cells essentially "eat" their damaged or unnecessary components. This not only eliminates cellular waste but also recycles the valuable building blocks for new cell structures.

As we age, the efficiency of autophagy tends to decline, contributing to the accumulation of cellular debris and potentially leading to various age-related conditions. However, when autophagy is stimulated, it acts as a rejuvenating force, helping to trim down this cellular waste, much like pruning a plant encourages new growth. The benefits of autophagy extend to various aspects of your health.

Autophagy is a fundamental process that plays a central role in maintaining cellular health and promoting longevity. It's a silent yet incredibly efficient janitor who works behind the scenes to ensure your cells are free from waste and damage. By facilitating the removal of cellular debris and recycling essential components, autophagy contributes to better skin, increased energy, and enhanced cognitive function.

Understanding the science of autophagy is an exciting journey, as it's still a field of research with much to uncover. However, autophagy has a significant role in how our bodies age, and by embracing intermittent fasting, you're not merely pursuing weight loss but also sitting at the table with the potential for a longer, more vibrant life

The implications of autophagy for anti-aging and overall health are profound, and it underscores the importance of lifestyle choices that support this process. By maintaining a balanced, nutritious diet and incorporating intermittent fasting, you're actively participating in this cellular clean-up, revitalizing your body and nurturing the promise of a more youthful and energetic you. Autophagy is your body's maintenance plan for your most cherished possession – your health. It's time to appreciate and support the silent janitor of your body as it works tirelessly to keep you in your best shape, both inside and out.

Aging is an inevitable part of life, and while the wisdom and experience that come with it are valuable treasures, the physical manifestations of aging are less welcome. We've all heard the saying, "Age is just a number," science reveals the truth behind this age-old adage. One of the most exciting developments in the quest for the elusive fountain of youth is the discovery of autophagy. This cellular process offers profound anti-aging benefits. In the following discussion, we will uncover the fascinating role of autophagy in maintaining youthfulness and promoting longevity, shedding light on how you can harness its potential for a more vibrant, youthful you.

ADVANCED STRATEGIES AND LONGEVITY

Autophagy, derived from the Greek words "auto" (self) and "phagy" (eating), is a cellular mechanism akin to an internal cleaning crew. It operates within your body to clean up and recycle damaged or unnecessary cellular components. Think of it as a meticulous janitor working tirelessly behind the scenes, ensuring that the factory of your cells functions optimally. Autophagy identifies and eliminates cellular waste while recycling valuable materials to build new, healthy structures.

As you age, the efficiency of autophagy naturally diminishes, leading to the accumulation of cellular debris and potentially contributing to the aging process. This debris buildup can manifest in various ways, from decreased skin elasticity to reduced energy levels and cognitive function. However, when autophagy is stimulated through specific practices such as intermittent fasting, it becomes a powerful anti-aging tool. By promoting cellular clean-up, autophagy effectively trims the cellular waste, encouraging a more youthful and vibrant version of yourself.

Autophagy is not merely a cellular process; it is a critical player in anti-aging. It presents an exciting avenue for maintaining a youthful appearance, high energy levels, and sharp cognitive function. As we delve into the science behind autophagy, we find that it holds significant potential to slow down the aging process and enhance our overall well-being.

The practical implications of this discovery are vast. By embracing lifestyle choices that promote autophagy, such as intermittent fasting and maintaining a nutrient-rich diet, you can actively engage with the anti-aging benefits of this cellular process. It's not about turning back the clock but embracing the present with vitality and a sense of timelessness.

Autophagy serves as a testament to the intricate and harmonious nature of our bodies. It's a reminder that we can influence our aging journey positively, allowing us to appreciate the wisdom of age while radiating the energy and vibrancy of youth. Embrace the potential of autophagy and the anti-aging wonders it offers, and take proactive steps to unlock a more youthful and vibrant you. After all, age may be just a number, but with autophagy, it can also be a symbol of grace, health, and enduring beauty.

Embracing Intermittent Fasting for Longevity

The quest for longevity, an age-old human aspiration, continues to capture our collective imagination. We all desire not just a longer life but a life filled with vibrancy, health, and the grace that accompanies aging. While the elixir of immortality remains a mythical pursuit, science is unveiling a promising avenue for extending our health span – the period of life marked by wellness and vitality. This avenue is none other than intermittent fasting. This practice offers the potential to not only extend your lifespan but also infuse it with quality, energy, and resilience. In the following discussion, we will explore the fascinating connection between intermittent fasting and longevity, offering insights on embracing this lifestyle for a more enduring and thriving existence.

Intermittent fasting is not a modern trend but a practice stretching roots back through the annals of history. It has been embraced by various cultures, often for religious or spiritual reasons. Today, the scientific community is unraveling the profound effects of intermittent fasting on our biology, shedding light on its potential to extend our health span and promote longevity.

ADVANCED STRATEGIES AND LONGEVITY

Intermittent fasting isn't about prolonged deprivation or restrictive diets; it's a pattern of eating that alternates between periods of eating and fasting. The fasting periods can vary, and there are several popular methods, such as the 16/8 method, the 5:2 pattern, and the Eat-Stop-Eat approach. What all these methods have in common is the power to stimulate autophagy, the cellular clean-up process we discussed earlier, and to enhance metabolic health. In conclusion, embracing intermittent fasting as a lifestyle choice holds the promise of extending your lifespan while enriching your healthspan. By incorporating intermittent fasting into your routine, you can tap into your body's innate ability to regenerate, repair, and thrive. It's not about rigid dieting but adopting a flexible approach to nourishing your body and mind.

The practical implications of intermittent fasting for longevity are both compelling and accessible. Intermittent fasting allows you to harmonize your body's natural rhythms, improve metabolic health, and stimulate the process of autophagy. This combination sets the stage for a life that isn't merely longer but filled with energy, vitality, and resilience.

As we navigate the intriguing intersection of science and age-old wisdom, we realize that the path to longevity is within our grasp. It's a journey that involves savoring the present, nurturing your health, and embracing the potential for a life that endures and flourishes. Intermittent fasting is a powerful ally on this journey, offering the prospect of a timeless existence marked by health and well-being. As you consider embracing intermittent fasting, remember that it's not about adding years to your life; it's about adding life to your years. With this practice, you're not merely extending your longevity. Still, you're also rewriting the story of your life with vitality, purpose, and enduring health.

Wrapping up this chapter and feeling like we've just finished a hearty meal of knowledge, we can sit back and savor it. Combining exercise with fasting can help us stay vibrant, and focusing on long-term maintenance ensures this is not a fleeting hobby but a part of our lifestyle. And with autophagy, we're not just living longer; we're living better. This isn't about chasing youth; it's about embracing the maturity and wisdom of our years with a body that's as strong and capable as we are spirited. Intermittent fasting isn't the fountain of youth, but it's certainly a path to a healthier, more vivacious life. Let's carry these strategies with us, like a cherished cookbook, ready to be used daily to enhance our lives for years.

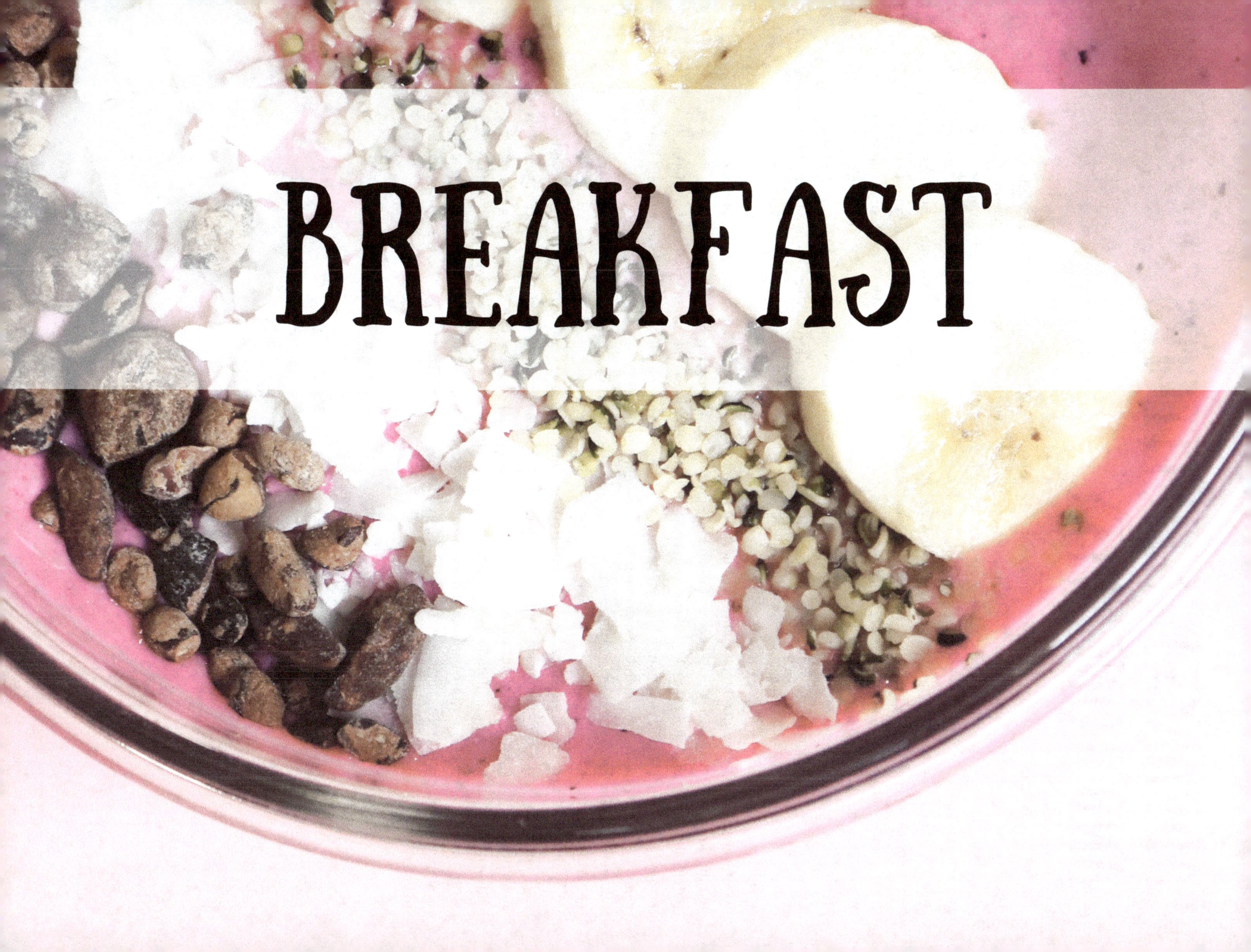
BREAKFAST

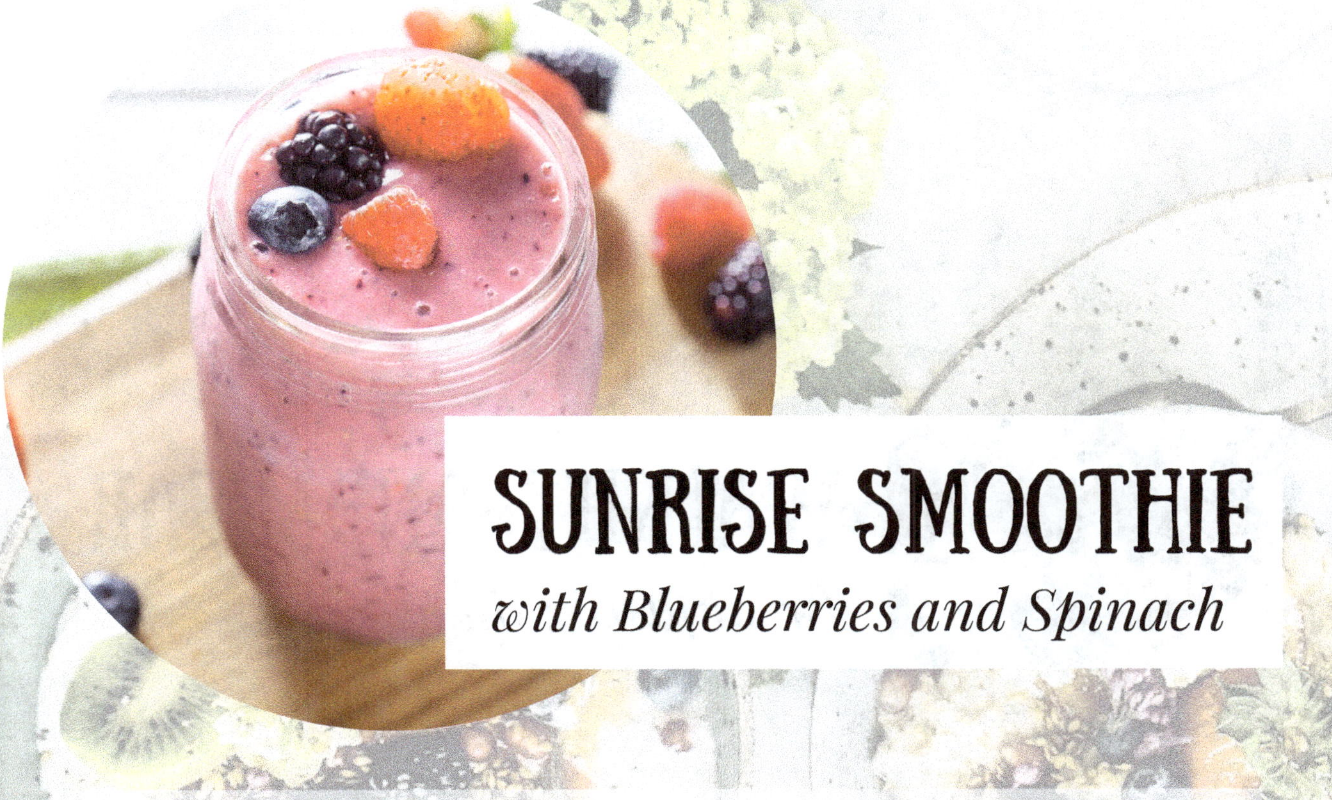

SUNRISE SMOOTHIE
with Blueberries and Spinach

Prep. Time: 5 minutes | **Cooking Time:** / | **Servings:** 2

INGREDIENTS

- ·1/2 cup fresh blueberries
- ·1 cup fresh spinach leaves
- ·1/2 banana
- ·1/2 cup unsweetened almond milk
- ·1/2 cup plain Greek yogurt
- ·1 tablespoon chia seeds
- ·1/2 teaspoon honey (optional)
- ·Ice cubes (optional)

DIRECTIONS

1. Wash the fresh blueberries and spinach leaves thoroughly.
2. Peel and slice the banana.
3. In a blender, add the fresh blueberries, spinach leaves, sliced banana, unsweetened almond milk, plain Greek yogurt, chia seeds, and honey (if desired).
4. If you prefer a colder smoothie, add a few ice cubes to the blender.
5. Blend all the ingredients until smooth and creamy, typically for about 1–2 minutes.
6. Check the consistency of the smoothie; if it's too thick, you can add more almond milk to reach your desired thickness.
7. Pour the Sunrise Smoothie into a glass and serve immediately.

NUTRITIONAL FACTS

Calories: 250 kcal Fat: 6g Protein: 12g Carbs: 42g Sugar: 23g Fiber: 8g Vitamin C: 34% DV Vitamin A: 57% DV Calcium: 34% DV Iron: 11% DV.

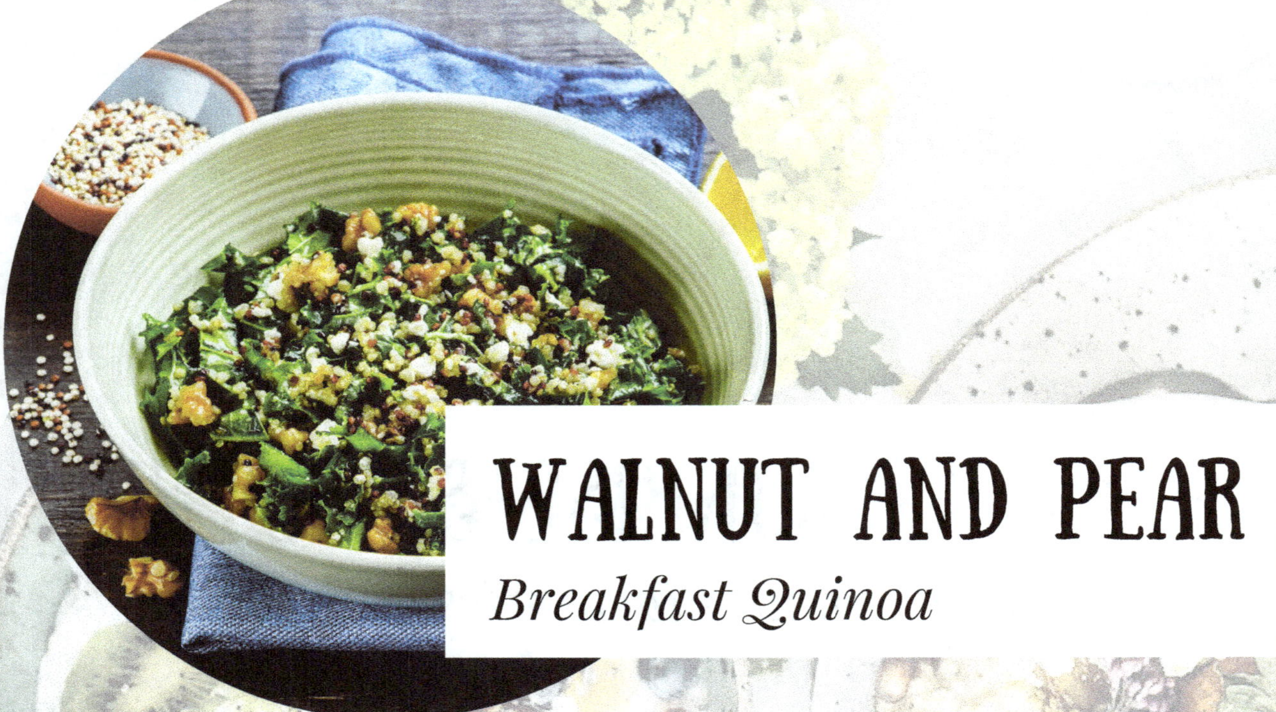

WALNUT AND PEAR
Breakfast Quinoa

Prep. Time: 10 minutes | **Cooking Time:** 15 minutes | **Servings:** 2

INGREDIENTS

- 1/2 cup quinoa
- 1 cup unsweetened almond milk
- 1 pear, ripe and diced
- 1/4 cup chopped walnuts
- 1/2 teaspoon ground cinnamon
- 1/4 teaspoon vanilla extract
- 1 tablespoon honey (optional)
- Fresh mint leaves for garnish (optional)

DIRECTIONS

1. Rinse the quinoa thoroughly in a fine-mesh strainer under cold running water.
2. In a saucepan, combine the rinsed quinoa and unsweetened almond milk. Bring to a boil over medium-high heat.
3. Once it reaches a boil, reduce the heat to low, cover the saucepan, and let it simmer for about 12-15 minutes, or until the quinoa is cooked and the liquid is absorbed. Stir occasionally to prevent sticking.
4. While the quinoa is cooking, dice the ripe pear and chop the walnuts.
5. Once the quinoa is cooked, remove it from heat and fluff it with a fork.
6. Stir in the diced pear, chopped walnuts, ground cinnamon, and vanilla extract. Mix well to combine.
7. If desired, drizzle with honey for added sweetness.
8. Divide the Walnut and Pear Breakfast Quinoa into two serving bowls.
9. Garnish with fresh mint leaves (optional) for a burst of flavor.
10. Serve warm, and enjoy your nutritious breakfast!

NUTRITIONAL FACTS

Calories: 350 kcal per serving Fat: 12g Protein: 8g Carbs: 56g Sugar: 16g Fiber: 7g Calcium: 260mg (26% DV) Iron: 3.5mg (19% DV) Vitamin C: 6.5mg (11% DV) Potassium: 320mg (9% DV)

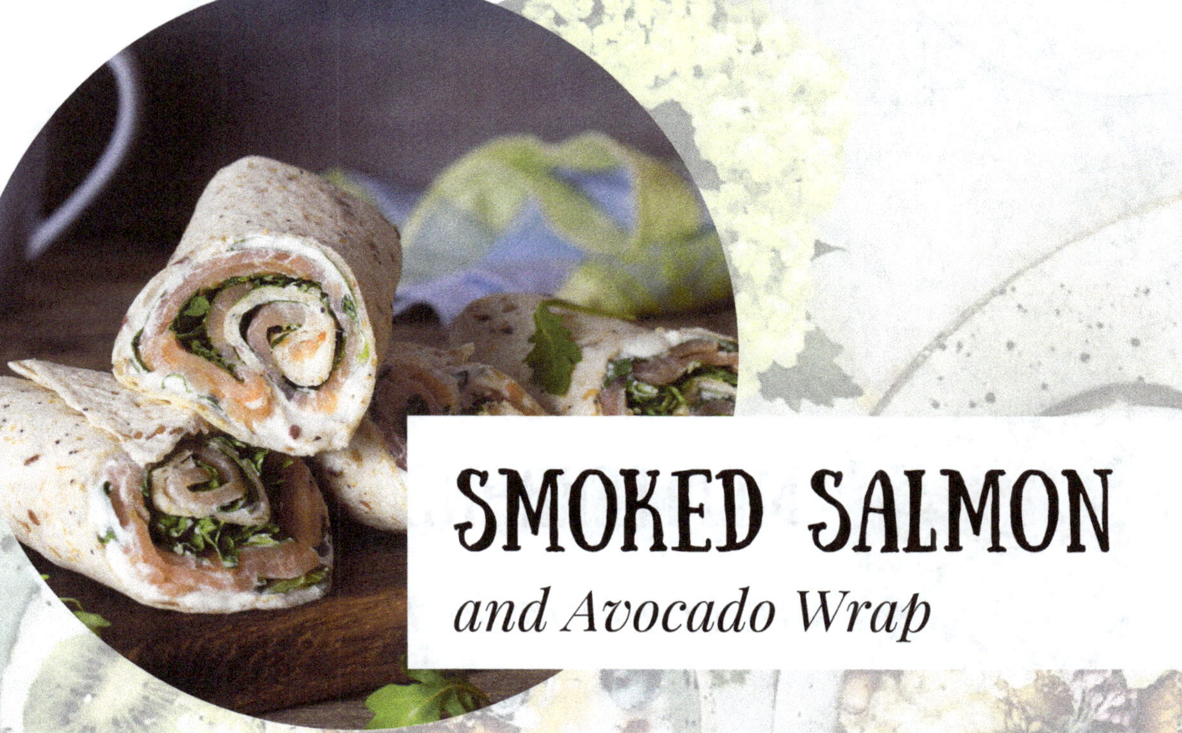

SMOKED SALMON
and Avocado Wrap

Prep. Time: 10 minutes | **Cooking Time:** / | **Servings:** 2

INGREDIENTS

- 4 large lettuce leaves (such as Romaine or iceberg)
- 4 oz smoked salmon
- 1 ripe avocado, sliced
- 1/2 cucumber, thinly sliced
- 1/4 red onion, thinly sliced
- 2 tablespoons Greek yogurt (low-fat)
- 1 teaspoon Dijon mustard
- 1/2 lemon, juiced
- Salt and pepper to taste
- Fresh dill for garnish (optional)

DIRECTIONS

1. Wash and dry the lettuce leaves, then set them aside.
2. Lay out a clean surface, such as a cutting board or parchment paper, to assemble the wraps.
3. On each lettuce leaf, place 1 oz of smoked salmon.
4. Add a few slices of ripe avocado on top of the smoked salmon.
5. Next, layer on some thinly sliced cucumber and red onion.
6. In a small bowl, combine the Greek yogurt, Dijon mustard, lemon juice, salt, and pepper. Mix until well combined.
7. Drizzle the yogurt-mustard sauce over the ingredients in each wrap.
8. If desired, garnish with fresh dill for added flavor and presentation.
9. Carefully fold the lettuce leaves over the ingredients to create wraps.
10. Serve immediately and enjoy your Smoked Salmon and Avocado Wraps!

NUTRITIONAL FACTS

Calories: 220 kcal per serving Fat: 12g Protein: 13g Carbs: 15g Sugar: 3g Fiber: 7g Vitamin C: 15mg (25% DV) Vitamin K: 45mcg (56% DV) Folate: 45mcg (11% DV) Potassium: 550mg (16% DV)

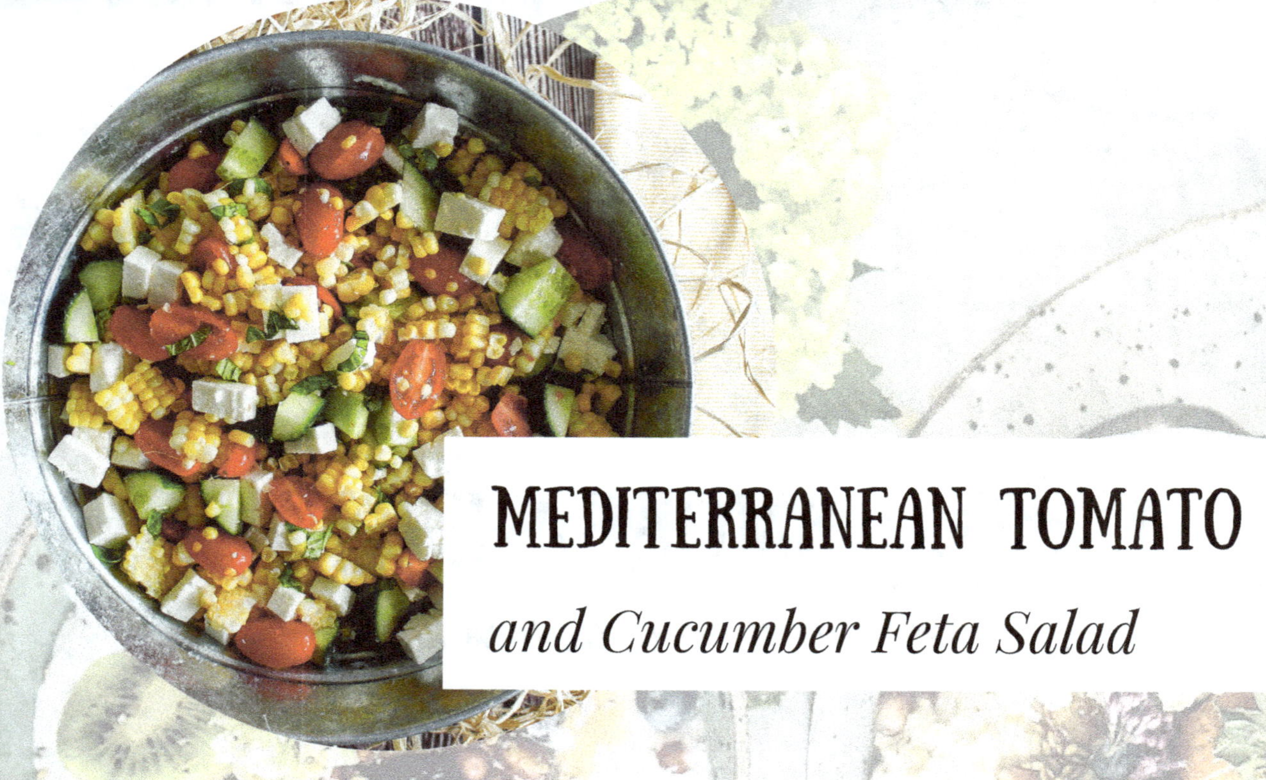

MEDITERRANEAN TOMATO
and Cucumber Feta Salad

Prep. Time: 5 minutes | **Cooking Time:** / | **Servings:** 4

INGREDIENTS

- ·4 cups cherry tomatoes, halved
- ·1 cucumber, diced
- ·1/2 red onion, thinly sliced
- ·1/2 cup crumbled feta cheese (reduced fat, if desired)
- ·1/4 cup Kalamata olives, pitted and sliced
- ·2 tablespoons extra-virgin olive oil
- ·1 tablespoon red wine vinegar
- ·1 teaspoon dried oregano
- ·Salt and pepper to taste
- ·Fresh basil leaves for garnish (optional)

DIRECTIONS

1. In a large salad bowl, combine the halved cherry tomatoes, diced cucumber, and thinly sliced red onion.
2. Add the crumbled feta cheese to the bowl.
3. Add the sliced Kalamata olives to the salad.
4. In a small bowl, whisk together the extra-virgin olive oil, red wine vinegar, dried oregano, salt, and pepper.
5. Drizzle the dressing over the salad ingredients in the large bowl.
6. Toss the salad to ensure all ingredients are well coated with the dressing.
7. If desired, garnish with fresh basil leaves for a burst of flavor and color.
8. Serve immediately as a refreshing and nutritious side dish or a light meal.

NUTRITIONAL FACTS

Calories: 175 kcal per serving Fat: 12g Protein: 4g Carbs: 13g Sugar: 7g Fiber: 3g Vitamin C: 28mg (47% DV) Vitamin K: 33mcg (41% DV) Calcium: 108mg (11% DV) Iron: 1mg (6% DV) Potassium: 406mg (12% DV)

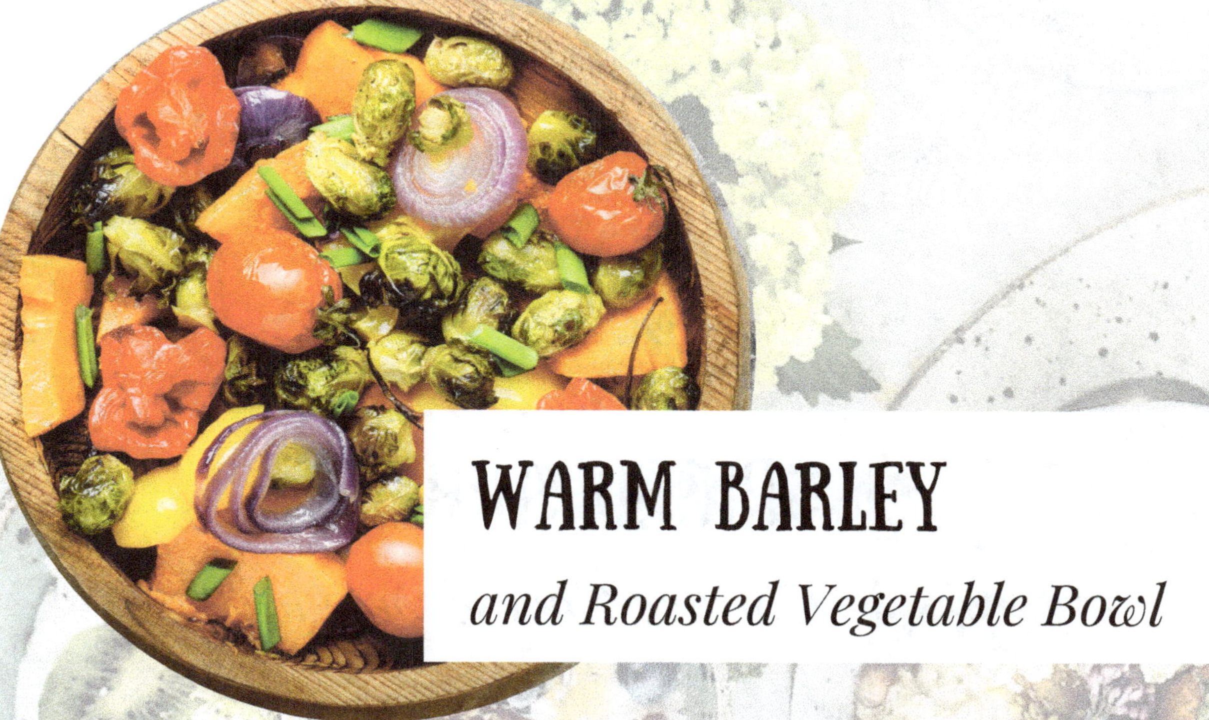

WARM BARLEY
and Roasted Vegetable Bowl

Prep. Time: 15 minutes | **Cooking Time:** 45 minutes | **Servings:** 4

INGREDIENTS

- 1 cup pearl barley
- 2 cups water
- 2 cups mixed vegetables (e.g., bell peppers, zucchini, cherry tomatoes, red onion)
- 2 tablespoons olive oil
- 1 teaspoon dried thyme
- Salt and pepper to taste
- 1/4 cup crumbled feta cheese (reduced-fat, if desired)
- 1/4 cup chopped fresh parsley
- 2 tablespoons balsamic vinegar
- 1 clove garlic, minced
- Lemon wedges for garnish (optional)

DIRECTIONS

1. Preheat your oven to 425°F (220°C).
2. Rinse the pearl barley in a fine-mesh strainer under cold running water.
3. In a saucepan, combine the rinsed pearl barley and 2 cups of water. Bring to a boil, then reduce the heat to low, cover, and simmer for 30-40 minutes or until the barley is tender and the water is absorbed. Remove from heat and fluff with a fork.
4. While the barley is cooking, prepare the roasted vegetables. Cut the mixed vegetables into bite-sized pieces and place them on a baking sheet.
5. Drizzle the olive oil over the vegetables, sprinkle with dried thyme, and season with salt and pepper. Toss to coat the vegetables evenly.
6. Roast the vegetables in the oven for 15-20 minutes or until tender and slightly caramelized. Stir them once or twice during roasting to ensure even cooking.
7. In a small bowl, whisk together the balsamic vinegar and minced garlic to create a dressing.
8. In a large mixing bowl, combine the cooked pearl barley, roasted vegetables, crumbled feta cheese, and chopped fresh parsley.
9. Drizzle the balsamic dressing over the barley and vegetable mixture, then gently toss to combine.
10. Serve the Warm Barley and Roasted Vegetable Bowls in individual serving dishes.
11. If desired, garnish with lemon wedges for an extra burst of flavor.

NUTRITIONAL FACTS

Calories: 270 kcal per serving Fat: 8g Protein: 7g Carbs: 45g Sugar: 5g Fiber: 8g Vitamin C: 24mg (40% DV) Vitamin A: 1490 IU (30% DV) Calcium: 107mg (11% DV) Iron: 2mg (11% DV) Potassium: 275mg (8% DV)

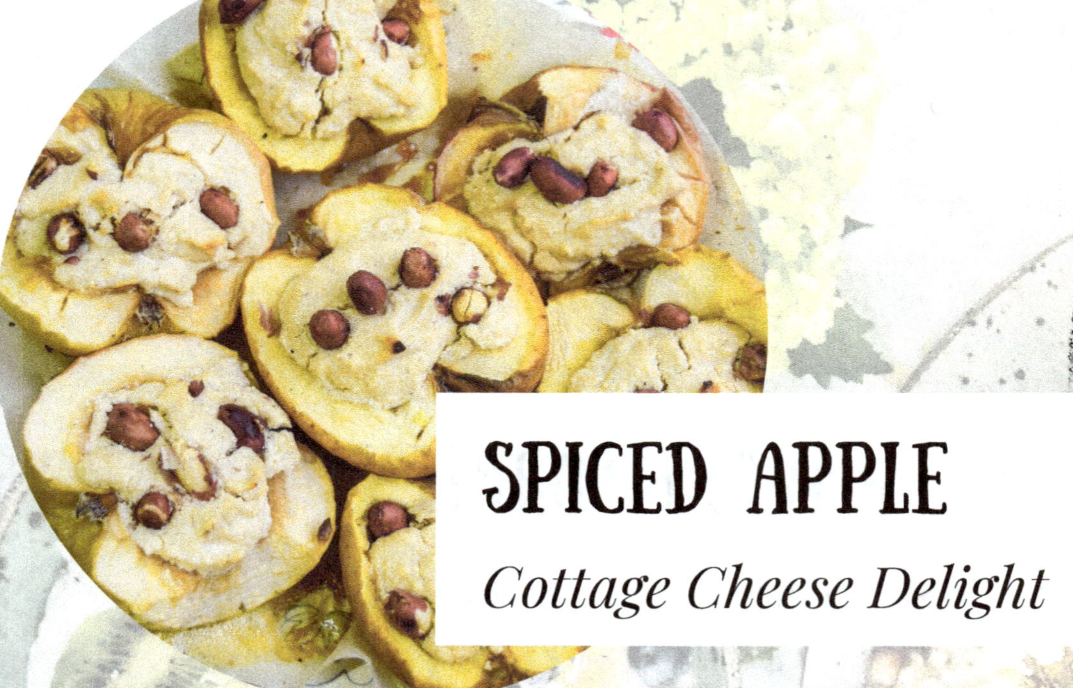

SPICED APPLE
Cottage Cheese Delight

Prep. Time: 10 minutes | **Cooking Time:** / | **Servings:** 2

INGREDIENTS

- 1 cup low-fat cottage cheese
- 2 medium apples, diced (choose a sweet variety)
- 1/2 teaspoon ground cinnamon
- 1/4 teaspoon ground nutmeg
- 1/4 teaspoon vanilla extract
- 2 tablespoons chopped walnuts
- 2 tablespoons honey (optional for drizzling)
- Fresh mint leaves for garnish (optional)

DIRECTIONS

1. In a mixing bowl, combine the low-fat cottage cheese, diced apples, ground cinnamon, ground nutmeg, and vanilla extract.
2. Gently stir the ingredients until the spices are evenly distributed and the apples are coated with the cinnamon and nutmeg.
3. Divide the spiced cottage cheese and apple mixture into two serving bowls.
4. Sprinkle chopped walnuts evenly over each bowl for added crunch and flavor.
5. If desired, drizzle honey over the top for a touch of sweetness.
6. Garnish with fresh mint leaves for a pop of color and freshness (optional).
7. Serve your Spiced Apple Cottage Cheese Delight immediately.

NUTRITIONAL FACTS

Calories: 250 kcal per serving Fat: 7g Protein: 15g Carbs: 36g Sugar: 26g Fiber: 5g Vitamin C: 10mg (17% DV) Calcium: 126mg (13% DV) Iron: 1mg (6% DV) Potassium: 316mg (9% DV)

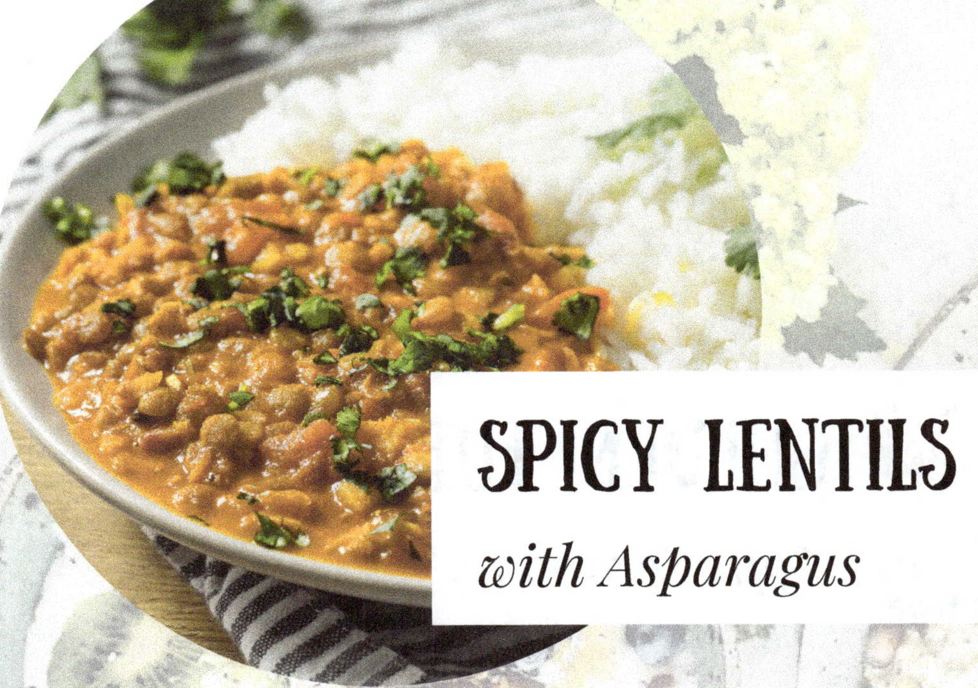

SPICY LENTILS
with Asparagus

Prep. Time: 10 minutes | **Cooking Time:** 20 minutes | **Servings:** 2

INGREDIENTS

- 1 cup brown lentils, rinsed and drained
- 2 cups water
- 1 bunch asparagus spears, trimmed and cut into 1-inch pieces
- 1/2 small onion, finely chopped
- 2 cloves garlic, minced
- 1 tablespoon olive oil
- 1/2 teaspoon ground cumin
- 1/2 teaspoon smoked paprika
- Salt and pepper to taste
- 2 large eggs
- Fresh parsley leaves for garnish (optional)

DIRECTIONS

1. In a medium saucepan, combine the rinsed brown lentils and 2 cups of water. Bring to a boil over high heat.
2. Reduce the heat to low, cover the saucepan, and simmer the lentils for about 20 minutes or until tender but still slightly firm. Drain any excess water and set the cooked lentils aside.
3. While the lentils are cooking, heat olive oil in a skillet over medium heat.
4. Add the chopped onion and cook for about 3-4 minutes until it becomes translucent.
5. Stir in the minced garlic and cook for 30 seconds until fragrant.
6. Add the asparagus pieces to the skillet and cook for 5-7 minutes or until tender and slightly caramelized.
7. Season the asparagus with ground cumin, smoked paprika, salt, and pepper. Stir to coat evenly.
8. Add the cooked lentils to the skillet with the asparagus and onion. Stir everything together and cook for 2-3 minutes to heat through.
9. In a separate pan, fry two large eggs to your preferred level of doneness (e.g., sunny-side-up or over-easy).
10. Divide the Savory Breakfast Lentils with Asparagus mixture into two serving bowls.
11. Place a fried egg on top of each bowl.
12. If desired, garnish with fresh parsley leaves for added flavor and presentation.
13. Serve immediately and enjoy your savory and protein-rich breakfast!

NUTRITIONAL FACTS

Calories: 330 kcal per serving Fat: 10g Protein: 18g Carbs: 42g Sugar: 4g Fiber: 18g Vitamin C: 10mg (17% DV) Iron: 6mg (33% DV) Folate: 275mcg (69% DV) Potassium: 720mg (21% DV)

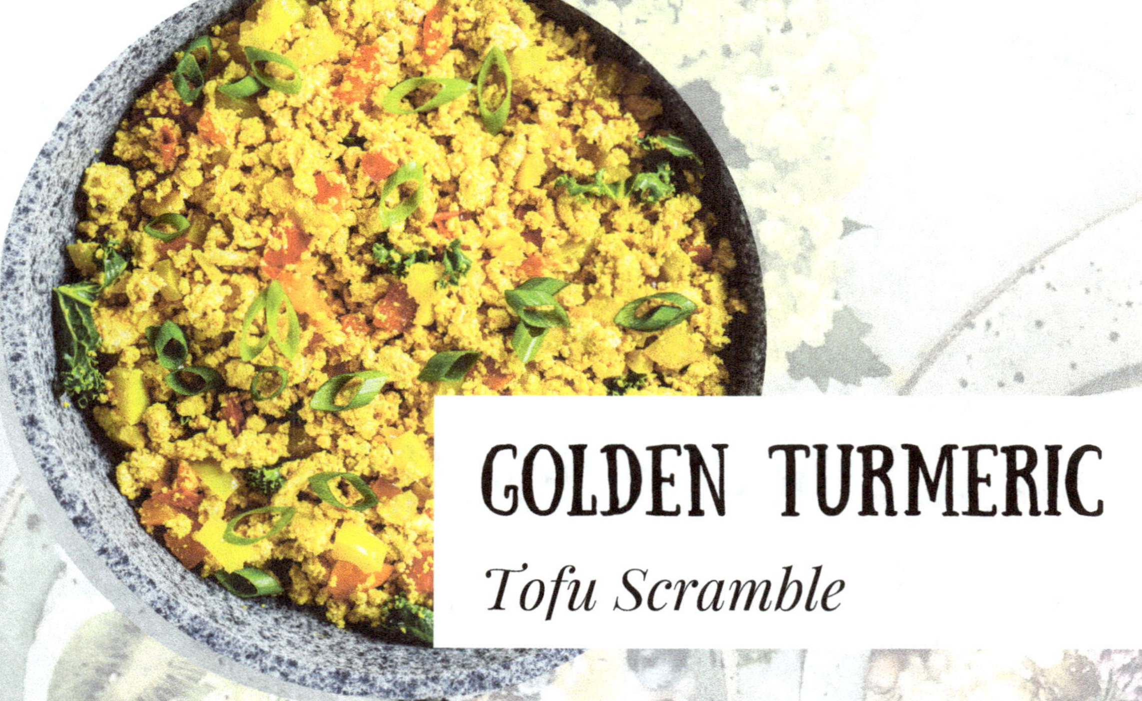

GOLDEN TURMERIC
Tofu Scramble

Prep. Time: 10 minutes | **Cooking Time:** 15 minutes | **Servings:** 2

INGREDIENTS

- 14 oz firm tofu, crumbled
- 1/2 teaspoon ground turmeric
- 1/2 teaspoon ground cumin
- 1/4 teaspoon ground paprika
- 1/4 teaspoon ground black salt (kala namak, for an eggy flavor)
- 1/4 teaspoon ground black pepper
- 1 tablespoon olive oil
- 1/2 small onion, finely chopped
- 1/2 red bell pepper, diced
- 1/2 cup cherry tomatoes, halved
- 2 cups fresh spinach leaves
- 2 tablespoons nutritional yeast (optional for added flavor)
- Fresh cilantro leaves for garnish (optional)

DIRECTIONS

1. Start by crushing the firm tofu in a bowl. Use your hands to crumble it into small pieces that resemble scrambled eggs.
2. In a small bowl, combine the ground turmeric, ground cumin, ground paprika, ground black salt (kala namak), and ground black pepper. Mix well to create a spice blend.
3. Heat olive oil in a large skillet over medium–high heat.
4. Add the finely chopped onion and sauté for about 2–3 minutes until it becomes translucent.
5. Stir in the diced red bell pepper and sauté for an additional 2–3 minutes until it starts to soften.
6. Add the cherry tomatoes to the skillet and cook for 2 minutes until they soften.
7. Add the crumbled tofu to the skillet, and sprinkle the spice blend over the tofu. Stir everything together to distribute the spices.
8. Cook the tofu scramble for about 5–7 minutes, stirring occasionally, until the tofu is heated through and lightly browned.
9. Stir in the fresh spinach leaves and cook for another 1–2 minutes until they wilt.
10. If desired, sprinkle nutritional yeast over the tofu scramble and stir to incorporate for added flavor.
11. Remove the skillet from heat.
12. Garnish with fresh cilantro leaves for an extra flavor and color (optional).
13. Serve your Golden Turmeric Tofu Scramble hot, and enjoy!

NUTRITIONAL FACTS

Calories: 280 kcal per serving Fat: 16g Protein: 24g Carbs: 15g Sugar: 4g Fiber: 5g Vitamin C: 59mg (99% DV)
Calcium: 276mg (28% DV) Iron: 6mg (34% DV) Potassium: 615mg (18% DV)

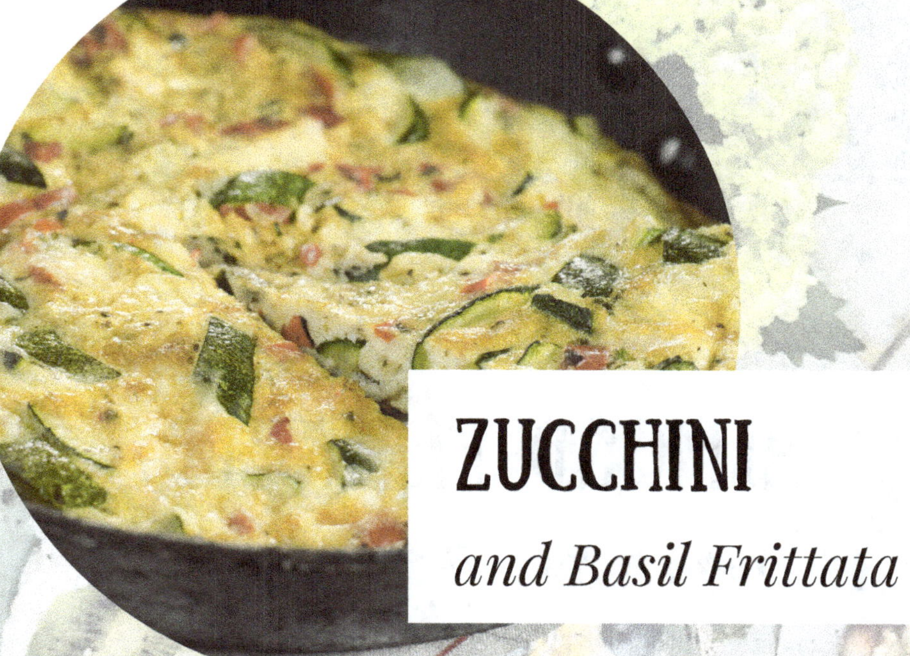

ZUCCHINI
and Basil Frittata

Prep. Time: 15 minutes | **Cooking Time:** 20 minutes | **Servings:** 4

INGREDIENTS

- ·6 large eggs
- ·2 medium zucchinis, thinly sliced
- ·1/2 cup diced red bell pepper
- ·1/2 cup diced onion
- ·1/2 cup fresh basil leaves, chopped
- ·1/2 cup grated Parmesan cheese
- ·2 tablespoons olive oil
- ·Salt and pepper to taste

DIRECTIONS

1. Preheat your oven's broiler on low.
2. In a mixing bowl, whisk the eggs until well beaten. Add a pinch of salt and pepper to taste.
3. Heat olive oil in a large ovenproof skillet over medium-high heat.
4. Add the diced onion and sauté for 2-3 minutes until it becomes translucent.
5. Stir in the thinly sliced zucchinis and continue to cook for another 4-5 minutes until the zucchinis soften and turn slightly golden.
6. Add the diced red bell pepper to the skillet and sauté for 2 minutes until it becomes tender.
7. Lower the heat to medium-low and pour the beaten eggs evenly over the sautéed vegetables in the skillet.
8. Sprinkle the chopped fresh basil evenly over the eggs.
9. Cook without stirring for about 4-5 minutes until the edges of the frittata start to set.
10. Sprinkle the grated Parmesan cheese over the top of the frittata.
11. Transfer the skillet to the preheated oven and broil on low for 4-5 minutes, until the frittata is set and the top is golden brown.
12. Carefully remove the skillet from the oven (use oven mitts), and let it cool slightly.
13. Using a spatula, gently loosen the frittata from the sides of the skillet.
14. Slide the Zucchini and Basil Frittata onto a cutting board.
15. Slice into wedges and serve immediately.

NUTRITIONAL FACTS

Calories: 220 kcal per serving Fat: 15g Protein: 13g Carbs: 8g Sugar: 4g Fiber: 2g Vitamin C: 30mg (50% DV)

Calcium: 210mg (21% DV) Iron: 2mg (11% DV) Potassium: 405mg (12% DV)

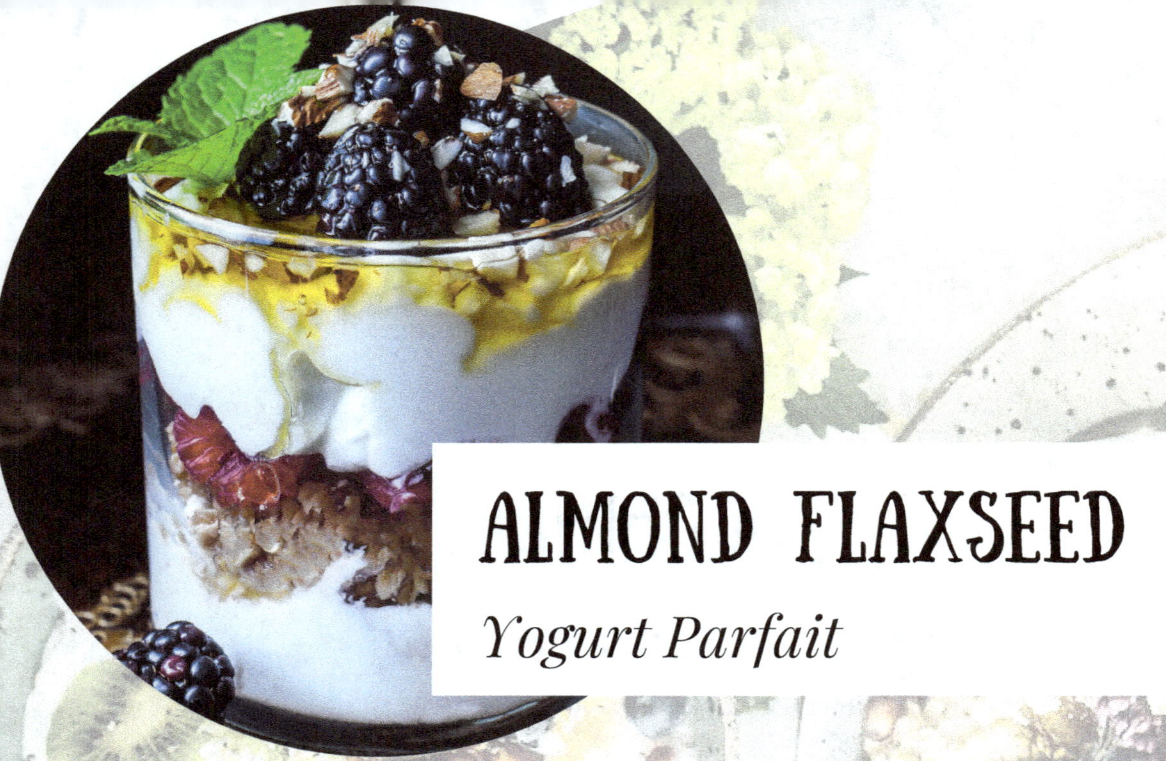

ALMOND FLAXSEED
Yogurt Parfait

Prep. Time: 10 minutes | **Cooking Time:** / | **Servings:** 2

INGREDIENTS

·1 cup low-fat Greek yogurt

·2 tablespoons almond butter

·2 tablespoons ground flaxseeds

·1 cup mixed berries (e.g., strawberries, blueberries, raspberries)

·1/4 cup chopped almonds

·1 tablespoon honey (optional)

·Fresh mint leaves for garnish (optional)

DIRECTIONS

1. In a small bowl, mix the almond butter with the low-fat Greek yogurt until well combined.
2. In two serving glasses or bowls, start layering your parfait. Begin with a spoonful of the almond-flavored yogurt at the bottom of each glass.
3. Sprinkle a layer of ground flaxseeds over the yogurt.
4. Add a layer of mixed berries on top of the flaxseeds.
5. Repeat the layering process until the glasses are filled, finishing with a layer of mixed berries on top.
6. If desired, drizzle honey over the top for added sweetness.
7. Sprinkle chopped almonds over the final berry layer for crunch and texture.
8. Garnish your Almond Flaxseed Yogurt Parfait with fresh mint leaves for a pop of color and freshness (optional).
9. Serve immediately and enjoy your delicious and nutrient-packed parfait!

NUTRITIONAL FACTS

Calories: 290 kcal per serving Fat: 14g Protein: 16g Carbs: 31g Sugar: 17g Fiber: 9g Vitamin C: 36mg (60% DV) Calcium: 280mg (28% DV) Iron: 2mg (11% DV) Potassium: 360mg (10% DV)

LUNCH

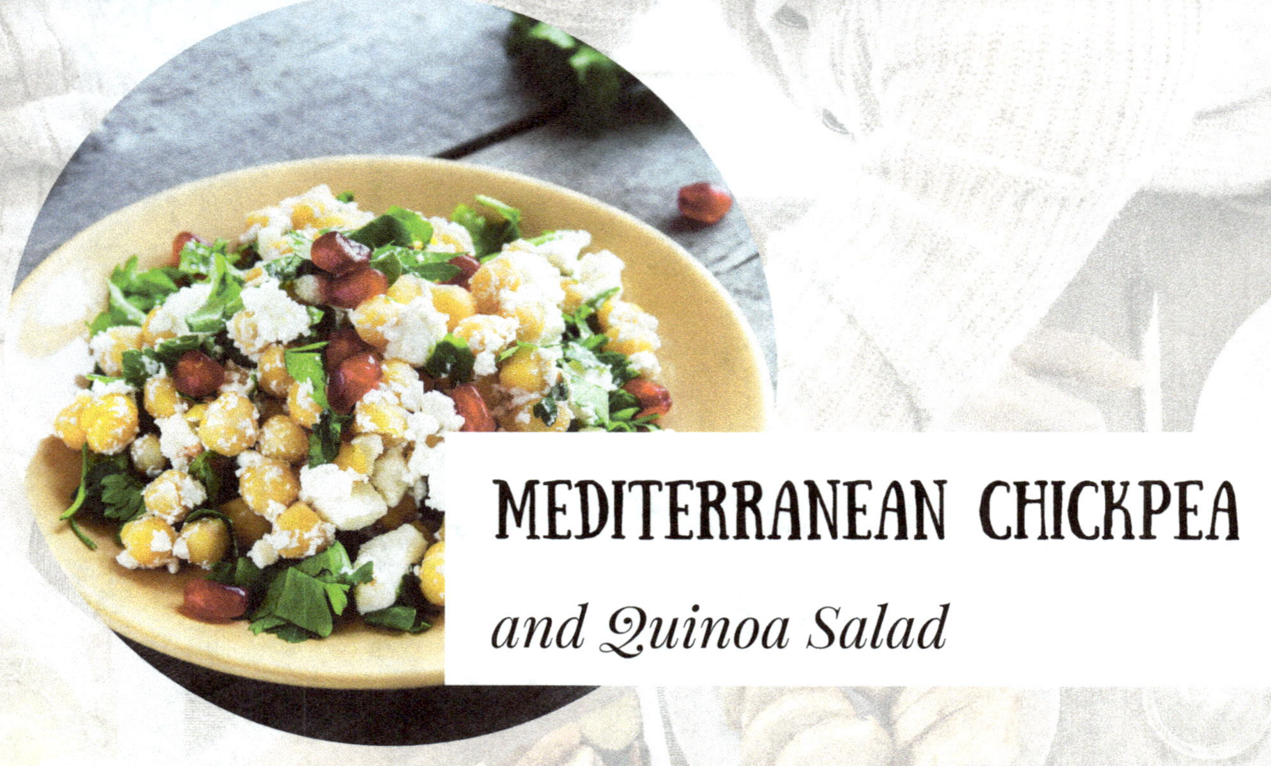

MEDITERRANEAN CHICKPEA
and *Quinoa Salad*

Prep. Time: 15 minutes | **Cooking Time:** 15 minutes | **Servings:** 4

INGREDIENTS

For the Salad:
- 1 cup cooked quinoa (cooled)
- 1 can (15 oz) chickpeas, drained and rinsed
- 1 cup cherry tomatoes, halved
- 1 cucumber, diced
- 1/2 red onion, finely chopped
- 1/4 cup Kalamata olives, pitted and sliced
- 1/4 cup fresh parsley, chopped
- 1/4 cup fresh mint leaves, chopped
- 1/2 cup crumbled feta cheese (optional)

For the Dressing:
- 3 tablespoons extra-virgin olive oil
- 2 tablespoons lemon juice
- 1 garlic clove, minced
- 1 teaspoon dried oregano
- Salt and black pepper to taste

DIRECTIONS

1. If you still need to cook the quinoa, rinse 1/2 cup of quinoa under cold water. In a saucepan, combine the rinsed quinoa with 1 cup of water. Bring to a boil, then reduce heat to low, cover, and simmer for about 15 minutes or until the quinoa is tender and the liquid is absorbed. Fluff with a fork and let it cool.

2. In a large salad bowl, combine the cooked and cooled quinoa, drained chickpeas, halved cherry tomatoes, diced cucumber, finely chopped red onion, sliced Kalamata olives, chopped fresh parsley, and chopped fresh mint leaves. If desired, add the crumbled feta cheese.

3. In a separate small bowl, whisk together the extra-virgin olive oil, lemon juice, minced garlic, dried oregano, salt, and black pepper to create the dressing.

4. Drizzle the dressing over the salad ingredients in the large bowl.

5. Toss all the ingredients until they are combined and coated with the dressing.

6. Taste and adjust the seasoning with additional salt, pepper, or lemon juice, if needed.

7. Let the Mediterranean Chickpea and Quinoa Salad sit for a few minutes to allow the flavors to meld.

8. Serve the salad in individual bowls or on plates.

9. Enjoy your nutritious and flavorful Mediterranean Chickpea and Quinoa Salad!

NUTRITIONAL FACTS

Calories: 350 kcal Fat: 14g Protein: 11g Carbs: 45g Sugar: 6g Fiber: 9g Vitamin C: 28mg (47% DV) Calcium: 125mg (13% DV) Iron: 3mg (17% DV) Potassium: 474mg (14% DV)

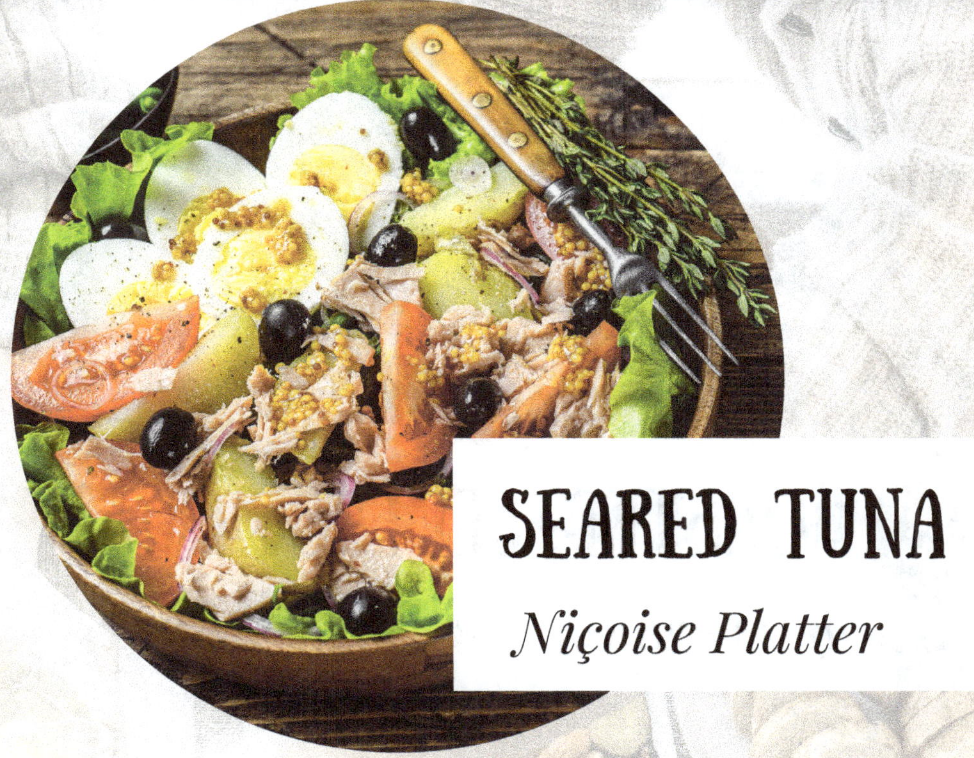

SEARED TUNA

Niçoise Platter

Prep. Time: 20 minutes | **Cooking Time:** 10 minutes | **Servings:** 4

INGREDIENTS

For the Tuna:
- 4 tuna steaks (about 6 oz each)
- 2 tablespoons olive oil
- Salt and black pepper to taste

For the Salad:
- 4 cups mixed salad greens (e.g., lettuce, arugula, spinach)
- 1 cup cherry tomatoes, halved
- 1 cup boiled and halved baby potatoes
- 1 cup blanched green beans, cut into bite-sized pieces
- 4 large eggs, hard-boiled and halved
- 1/4 cup Kalamata olives, pitted
- 2 tablespoons capers
- 1/4 cup red onion, thinly sliced

For the Dressing:
- 3 tablespoons extra-virgin olive oil
- 2 tablespoons red wine vinegar
- 1 teaspoon Dijon mustard
- 1 garlic clove, minced
- Salt and black pepper to taste

DIRECTIONS

1. Season the tuna steaks with salt and black pepper on both sides.
2. Heat 2 tablespoons of olive oil in a skillet or grill pan over high heat.
3. Once the oil is hot, add the tuna steaks to the skillet. Sear for about 2-3 minutes on each side for medium-rare or longer if you prefer your tuna more well-done.
4. Remove the seared tuna from the skillet and let it rest for a few minutes before slicing it into thin strips.
5. While the tuna is resting, prepare the salad components. On a large serving platter or individual plates, arrange the mixed salad greens, halved cherry tomatoes, boiled baby potatoes, blanched green beans, hard-boiled eggs, Kalamata olives, capers, and thinly sliced red onion.
6. In a small bowl, whisk together the extra-virgin olive oil, red wine vinegar, Dijon mustard, minced garlic, salt, and black pepper to make the dressing.
7. Drizzle the dressing over the salad ingredients.
8. Top the salad with the sliced seared tuna.
9. Serve the Seared Tuna Niçoise Platter immediately and enjoy!

NUTRITIONAL FACTS

Calories: 390 kcal Fat: 20g Protein: 30g Carbs: 24g Sugar: 4g Fiber: 4g Vitamin C: 29mg (48% DV) Calcium: 82mg (8% DV) Iron: 4mg (22% DV) Potassium: 824mg (23% DV)

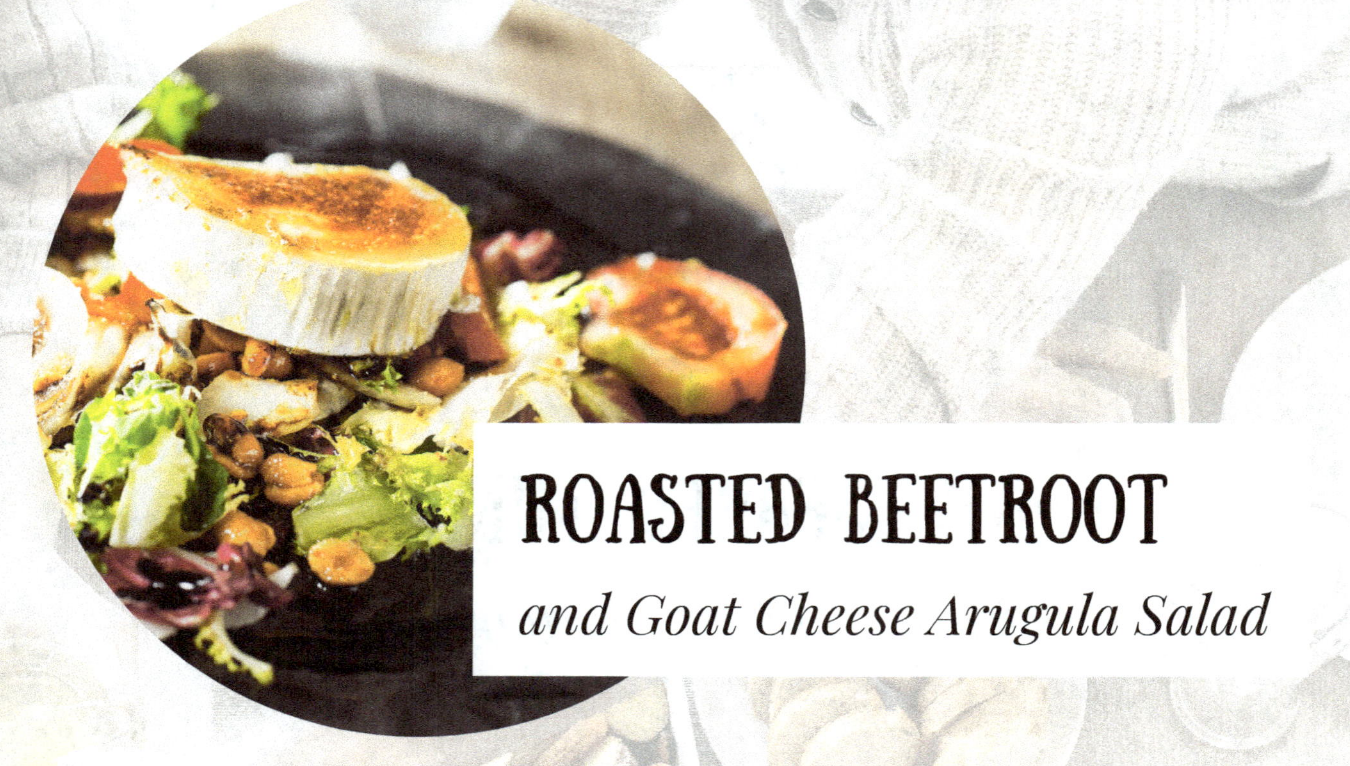

ROASTED BEETROOT
and Goat Cheese Arugula Salad

Prep. Time: 15 minutes | **Cooking Time:** 45 minutes | **Servings:** 4

INGREDIENTS

For the Salad:
- 4 medium-sized beetroots, peeled and cut into small wedges
- 4 cups fresh arugula
- 1/2 cup crumbled goat cheese
- 1/4 cup walnuts, toasted and chopped
- 1/4 cup red onion, thinly sliced
- 2 tablespoons fresh basil leaves, torn
- Salt and black pepper to taste

For the Dressing:
- 3 tablespoons extra-virgin olive oil
- 2 tablespoons balsamic vinegar
- 1 teaspoon honey
- 1 clove garlic, minced
- Salt and black pepper to taste

DIRECTIONS

1. Preheat your oven to 400°F (200°C).
2. Place the peeled and cut beetroot wedges on a baking sheet. Drizzle with olive oil, season with salt and black pepper, and toss to coat.
3. Roast the beetroot in the preheated oven for about 45 minutes or until they are tender when pierced with a fork. Remove from the oven and let them cool to room temperature.
4. While the beetroots are roasting, prepare the dressing. In a small bowl, whisk together the extra-virgin olive oil, balsamic vinegar, honey, minced garlic, salt, and black pepper. Set aside.
5. In a large serving bowl, arrange the fresh arugula.
6. Once the roasted beetroots have cooled, add them to the arugula in the serving bowl.
7. Scatter the crumbled goat cheese, toasted and chopped walnuts, thinly sliced red onion, and torn fresh basil leaves over the arugula and roasted beetroots.
8. Drizzle the dressing evenly over the salad.
9. Toss the salad gently to combine all the ingredients and coat them with the dressing.
10. Serve the Roasted Beetroot and Goat Cheese Arugula Salad immediately.

NUTRITIONAL FACTS

Calories: 225 kcal Fat: 15g Protein: 6g Carbs: 18g Sugar: 9g Fiber: 3g Vitamin C: 9mg (15% DV) Calcium: 75mg (8% DV) Iron: 2mg (11% DV) Potassium: 470mg (13% DV)

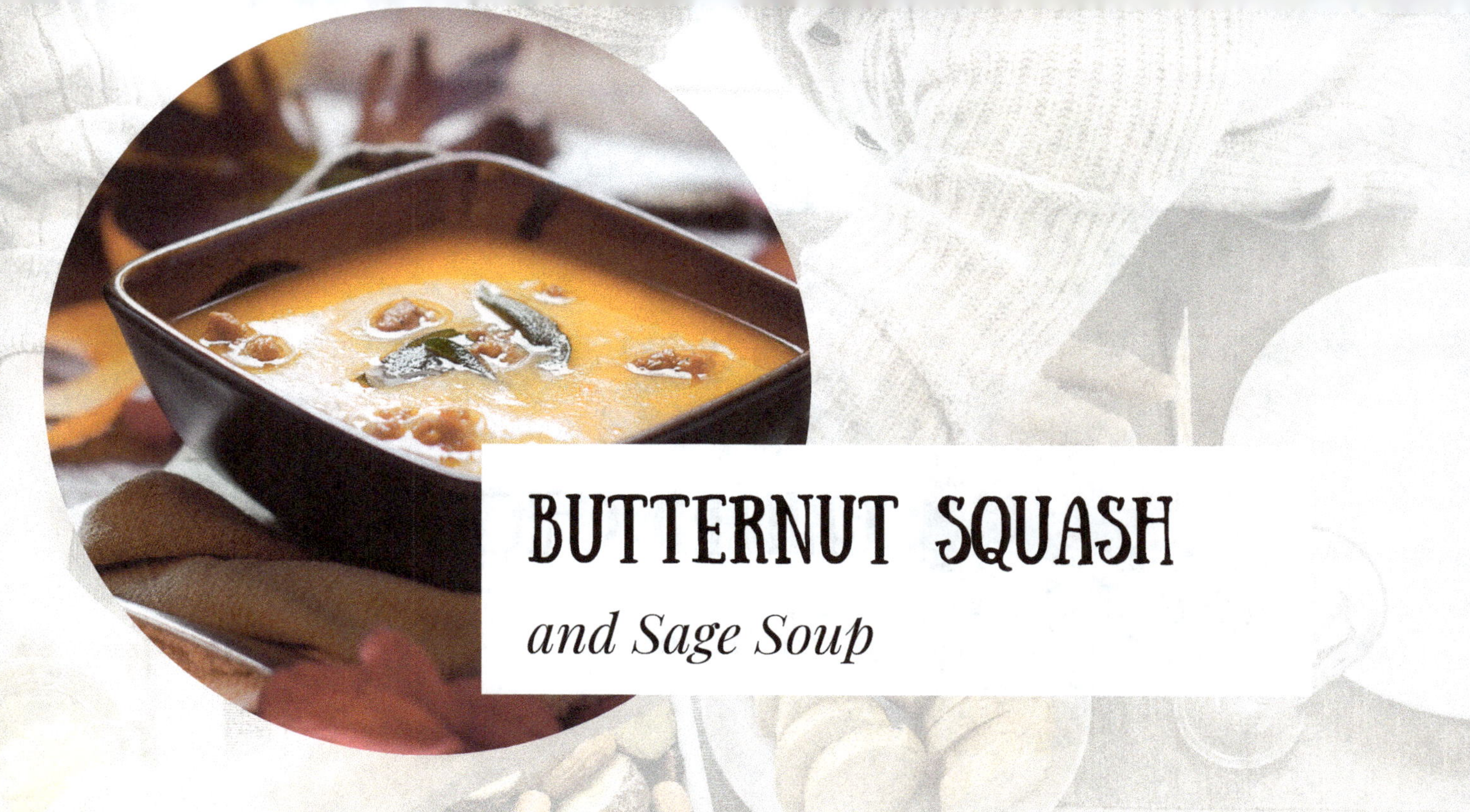

BUTTERNUT SQUASH
and Sage Soup

Prep. Time: 20 minutes | **Cooking Time:** 40 minutes | **Servings:** 6

INGREDIENTS

·1 medium-sized butternut squash (about 2 pounds), peeled, seeded, and cubed

·1 large onion, chopped

·2 cloves garlic, minced

·2 tablespoons olive oil

·4 cups vegetable broth (low-sodium)

·1/2 teaspoon dried sage (or 1 tablespoon fresh sage, chopped)

·Salt and black pepper to taste

·1/2 cup low-fat Greek yogurt (optional for garnish)

·Fresh sage leaves (optional, for garnish)

DIRECTIONS

1.   In a large soup pot, heat the olive oil over medium heat. Add the chopped onion and minced garlic. Sauté for about 5 minutes or until the onions become translucent.

2.   Add the cubed butternut squash and dried sage to the pot. Sauté for an additional 5 minutes, stirring occasionally.

3.   Pour in the vegetable broth, and bring the mixture to a boil. Reduce the heat to low, cover the pot, and simmer for 25-30 minutes or until the butternut squash is tender when pierced with a fork.

4.   Remove the pot from the heat and let it cool slightly.

5.   Using an immersion blender, carefully blend the soup until smooth and creamy. Alternatively, you can transfer the soup in batches to a regular blender, but be cautious with hot liquids.

6.   Return the blended soup to the pot and reheat it over low heat. Season with salt and black pepper to taste. Adjust the seasoning as needed.

7.   Serve the Butternut Squash and Sage Soup in bowls. If desired, garnish each bowl with a dollop of low-fat Greek yogurt and a few fresh sage leaves.

8.   Enjoy your delicious and comforting soup!

NUTRITIONAL FACTS

Calories: 120 kcal Fat: 4g Protein: 2g Carbs: 23g Sugar: 5g Fiber: 4g Vitamin A: 11,602 IU (232% DV) Vitamin C: 32mg (53% DV) Calcium: 87mg (9% DV) Iron: 1mg (6% DV) Potassium: 621mg (18% DV)

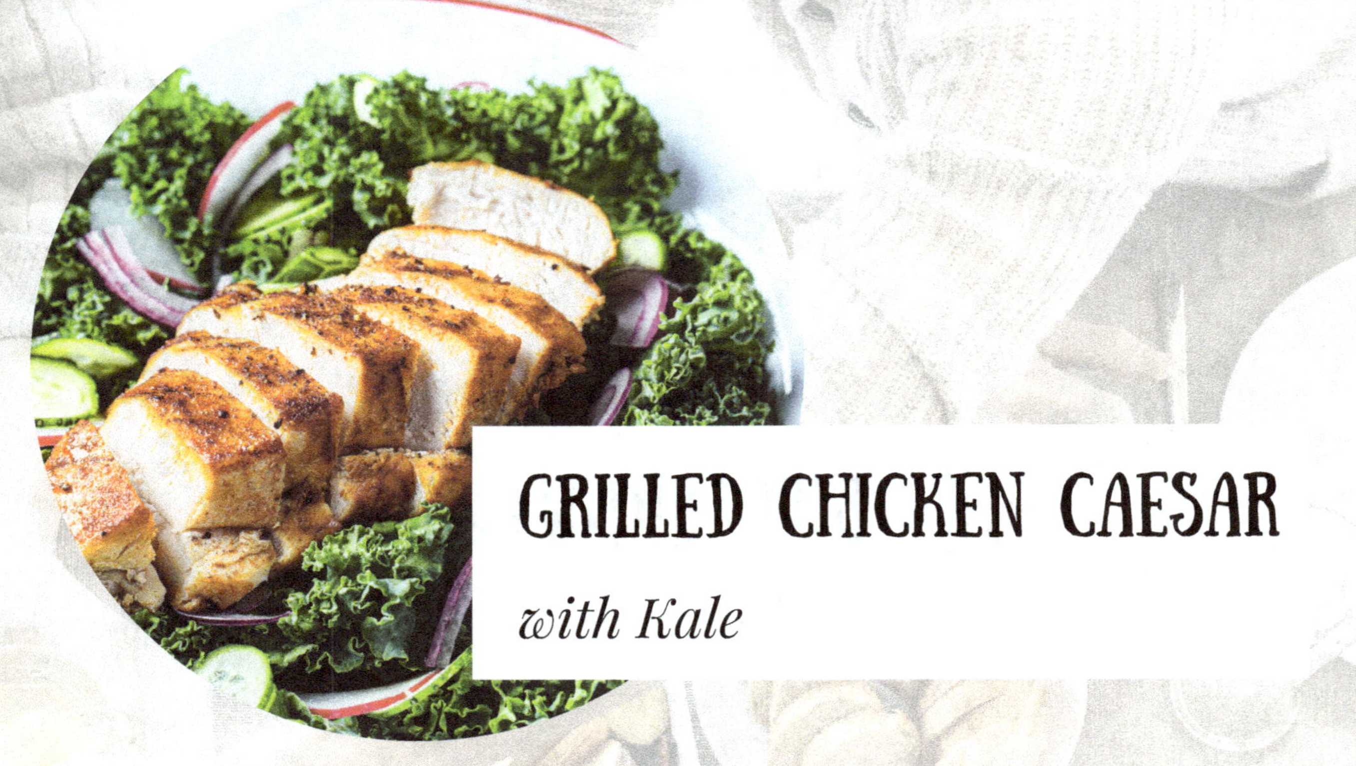

GRILLED CHICKEN CAESAR

with Kale

Prep. Time: 20 minutes | **Cooking Time:** 10 minutes | **Servings:** 4

INGREDIENTS

For the Salad:
- 4 boneless, skinless chicken breasts
- 1 tablespoon olive oil
- Salt and black pepper to taste
- 8 cups chopped kale leaves, stems removed
- 1 cup cherry tomatoes, halved
- 1/4 cup grated Parmesan cheese
- 1/4 cup whole wheat croutons

For the Caesar Dressing:
- 1/2 cup plain Greek yogurt
- 2 tablespoons grated Parmesan cheese
- 1 tablespoon lemon juice
- 1 clove garlic, minced
- 1 teaspoon Dijon mustard
- 1 teaspoon Worcestershire sauce
- Salt and black pepper to taste

DIRECTIONS

1. Preheat your grill to medium-high heat.
2. Brush the chicken breasts with olive oil and season them with salt and black pepper.
3. Grill the chicken breasts for about 5 minutes per side or until they are cooked and have excellent grill marks. The internal temperature should reach 165°F (74°C). Remove the chicken from the grill and let it rest for a few minutes before slicing.
4. While the chicken is resting, prepare the Caesar dressing. In a bowl, whisk together the plain Greek yogurt, grated Parmesan cheese, lemon juice, minced garlic, Dijon mustard, Worcestershire sauce, salt, and black pepper. Adjust the seasoning to your taste.
5. In a large salad bowl, combine the chopped kale leaves and cherry tomato halves.
6. Slice the grilled chicken breasts into thin strips and add them to the salad bowl.
7. Drizzle the Caesar dressing over the salad and toss everything together until the kale is well coated.
8. Top the salad with grated Parmesan cheese and whole wheat croutons.
9. Serve the Grilled Chicken Caesar with Kale immediately.

NUTRITIONAL FACTS

Calories: 290 kcal Fat: 10g Protein: 34g Carbs: 18g Sugar: 4g Fiber: 3g Vitamin A: 17322 IU (346% DV)

Vitamin C: 99mg (165% DV) Calcium: 271mg (27% DV) Iron: 2mg (11% DV) Potassium: 709mg (20% DV)

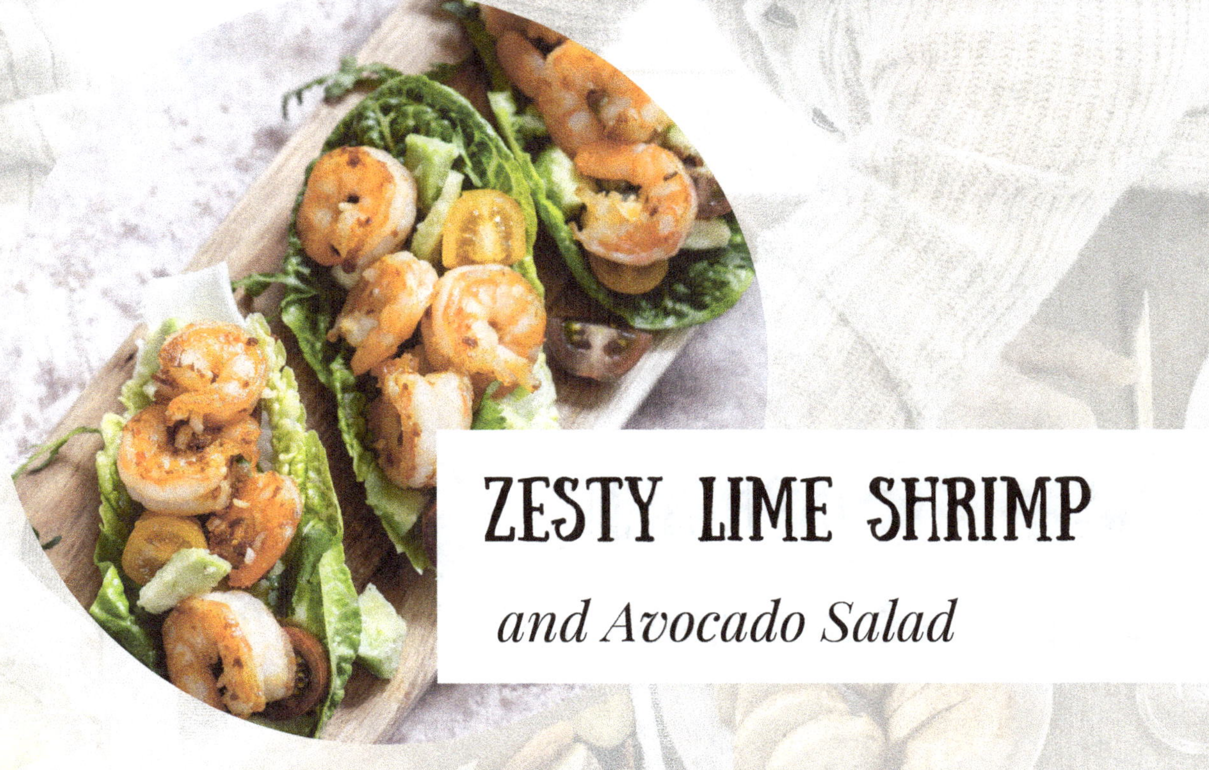

ZESTY LIME SHRIMP
and Avocado Salad

Prep. Time: 20 minutes | **Cooking Time:** 5 minutes | **Servings:** 4

INGREDIENTS

For the Lime Shrimp:
- 1 pound large shrimp, peeled and deveined
- 2 cloves garlic, minced
- 1 tablespoon olive oil
- Zest and juice of 2 limes
- Salt and black pepper to taste

For the Salad:
- 4 cups mixed greens (e.g., spinach, arugula, and romaine)
- 2 avocados, diced
- 1 cup cherry tomatoes, halved
- 1/4 cup red onion, finely chopped
- 1/4 cup fresh cilantro, chopped
- 1/4 cup crumbled feta cheese (optional)

For the Dressing:
- 2 tablespoons olive oil
- Zest and juice of 1 lime
- 1 teaspoon honey or maple syrup
- Salt and black pepper to taste

DIRECTIONS

1. In a bowl, combine the minced garlic, olive oil, lime zest, lime juice, salt, and black pepper. Mix well.
2. Place the peeled and deveined shrimp in a zip-top bag and pour the marinade over them. Seal the bag and gently massage to ensure the shrimp are evenly coated. Let them marinate for about 10 minutes.
3. While the shrimp are marinating, prepare the salad. In a large salad bowl, combine the mixed greens, diced avocados, cherry tomato halves, finely chopped red onion, and fresh cilantro. If desired, add crumbled feta cheese to the salad.
4. In a hot skillet or grill pan over medium-high heat, cook the marinated shrimp for about 2-3 minutes per side or until they turn pink and opaque. Be careful not to overcook them.
5. In a small bowl, whisk together the olive oil, lime zest, lime juice, honey or maple syrup, salt, and black pepper to create the dressing.
6. Drizzle the dressing over the salad and toss gently to combine.
7. Divide the salad onto serving plates and top each with the zesty lime shrimp.
8. Serve the Zesty Lime Shrimp and Avocado Salad immediately.

NUTRITIONAL FACTS

Calories: 350 kcal Fat: 22g Protein: 23g Carbs: 20g Sugar: 5g Fiber: 10g Vitamin A: 3522 IU (70% DV) Vitamin C: 33mg (55% DV) Calcium: 140mg (14% DV) Iron: 3mg (17% DV) Potassium: 813mg (23% DV)

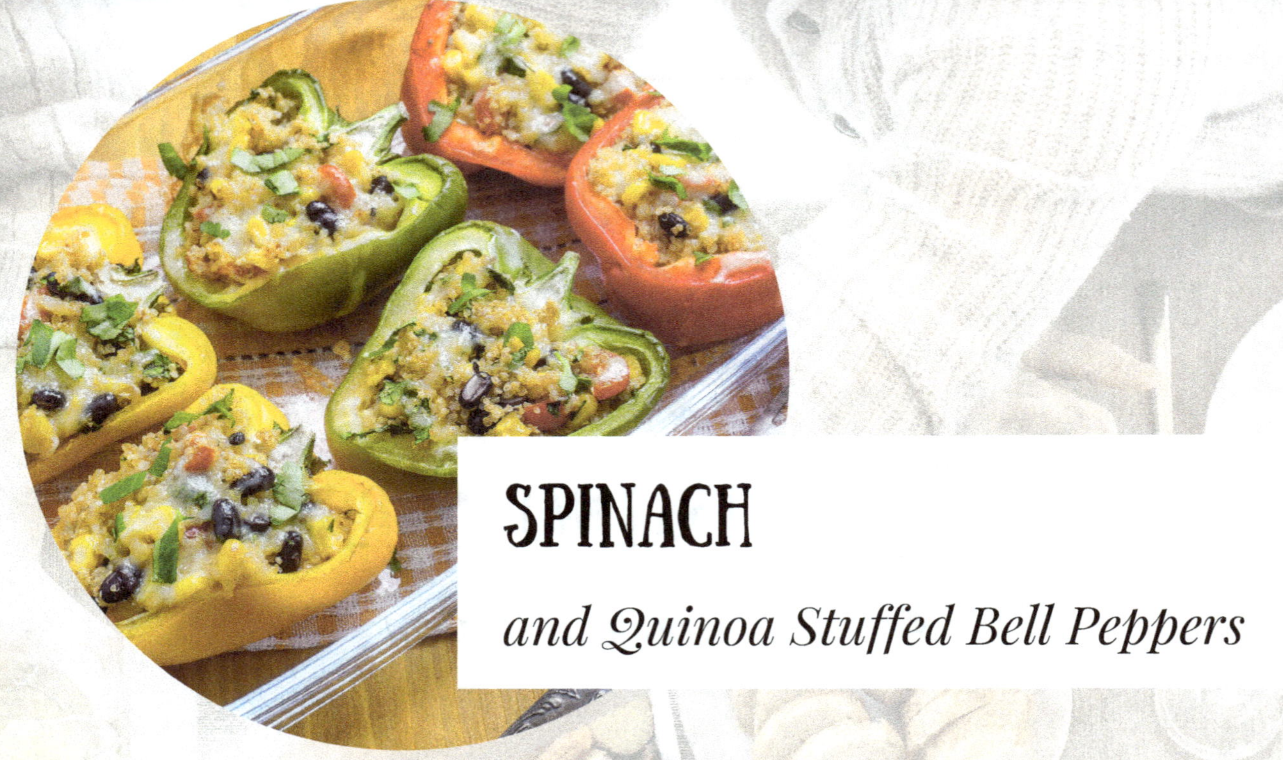

SPINACH
and Quinoa Stuffed Bell Peppers

Prep. Time: 20 minutes | **Cooking Time:** 35 minutes | **Servings:** 4

INGREDIENTS

- 4 large bell peppers, any color
- 1 cup quinoa, rinsed and drained
- 2 cups vegetable broth or water
- 1 tablespoon olive oil
- 1 onion, finely chopped
- 2 cloves garlic, minced
- 2 cups baby spinach, chopped
- 1 (14-ounce) can of diced tomatoes, drained
- 1 teaspoon dried oregano
- 1/2 teaspoon ground cumin
- Salt and black pepper to taste
- 1 cup shredded mozzarella cheese (optional, omit for a dairy-free version)
- Fresh basil leaves, for garnish (optional)

DIRECTIONS

1. Preheat your oven to 375°F (190°C).
2. Cut the tops off the bell peppers and remove the seeds and membranes. Rinse them and set them aside.
3. In a medium saucepan, combine the quinoa and vegetable broth or water. Bring to a boil, then reduce the heat to low, cover, and simmer for 15-20 minutes or until the quinoa is cooked and the liquid is absorbed. Remove from heat and fluff with a fork.
4. In a large skillet, heat the olive oil over medium heat. Add the chopped onion and cook for 3-4 minutes until it becomes translucent.
5. Add the minced garlic and cook for another 30 seconds until fragrant.
6. Stir in the chopped spinach and cook for 2-3 minutes until wilted.
7. Add the drained diced tomatoes, dried oregano, ground cumin, salt, and black pepper to the skillet. Cook for 2-3 minutes to heat through and combine the flavors.
8. Remove the skillet from heat and stir in the cooked quinoa. Mix everything together until well combined.
9. Stuff each bell pepper with the spinach and quinoa mixture, pressing down gently to pack the filling.
10. Place the stuffed bell peppers in a baking dish. If desired, sprinkle shredded mozzarella cheese on top of each stuffed pepper.
11. Cover the baking dish with aluminum foil and bake in the oven for 20-25 minutes or until the bell peppers are tender.
12. Remove the foil and bake for 5-10 minutes or until the cheese is melted and slightly golden.
13. Garnish with fresh basil leaves if desired.
14. Serve the Spinach and Quinoa Stuffed Bell Peppers hot, and enjoy!

NUTRITIONAL FACTS

Calories: 312 kcal Fat: 7g Protein: 11g Carbs: 54g Sugar: 8g Fiber: 9g Vitamin A: 10196 IU (204% DV) Vitamin C: 231mg (385% DV) Calcium: 158mg (16% DV) Iron: 4mg (22% DV) Potassium: 1054mg (30% DV)

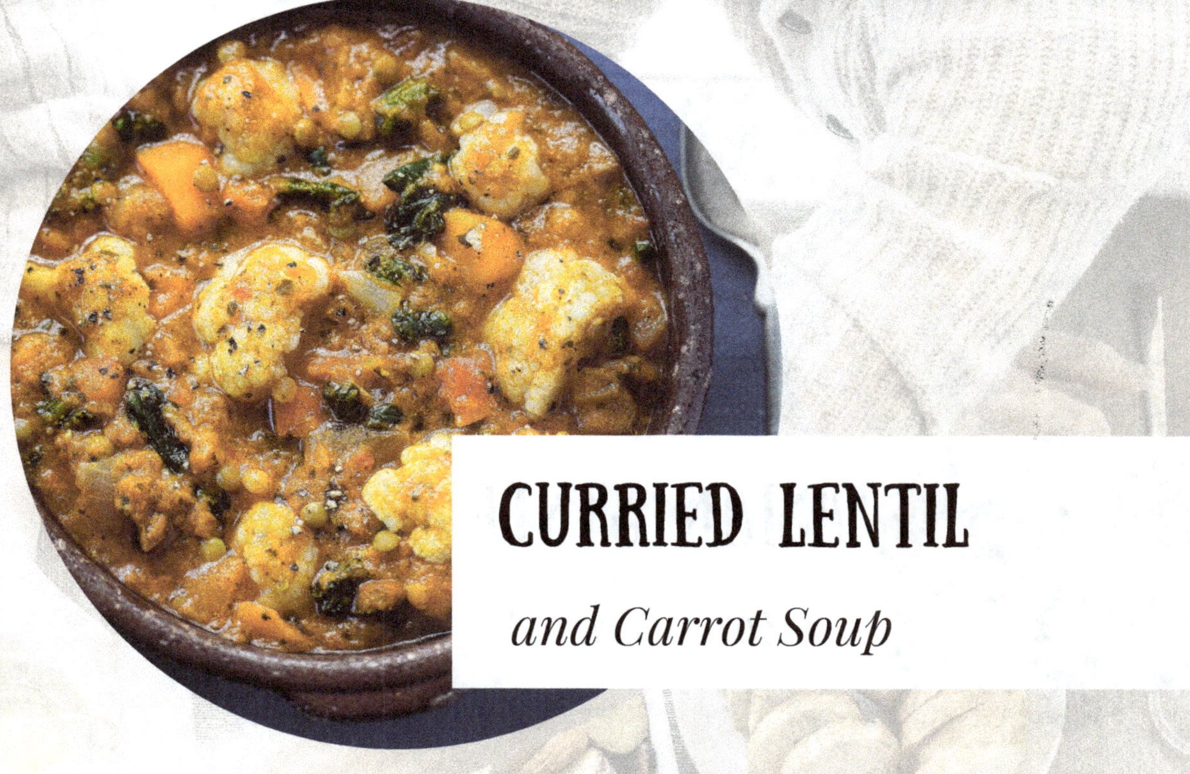

CURRIED LENTIL

and Carrot Soup

Prep. Time: 15 minutes | **Cooking Time:** 25 minutes | **Servings:** 4

INGREDIENTS

·1 cup red lentils, rinsed and drained
·4 cups vegetable broth
·2 cups carrots, peeled and chopped
·1 onion, chopped
·2 cloves garlic, minced
·1 tablespoon olive oil
·1 tablespoon curry powder
·1 teaspoon ground cumin
·1/2 teaspoon ground turmeric
·1/2 teaspoon ground coriander
·Salt and black pepper to taste
·1 (14-ounce) can diced tomatoes
·1 (14-ounce) can coconut milk
·Fresh cilantro leaves for garnish
(optional)
·Lime wedges for serving (optional)

DIRECTIONS

1.In a large pot, heat the olive oil over medium heat. Add the chopped onion and cook for 3-4 minutes until it becomes translucent.

2.Add the minced garlic and cook for another 30 seconds until fragrant.

3.Stir in the curry powder, ground cumin, turmeric, and coriander. Cook for 1-2 minutes to toast the spices and release their flavors.

4.Add the chopped carrots to the pot and cook for 2-3 minutes, stirring occasionally.

5.Pour in the vegetable broth and red lentils. Bring the mixture to a boil, then reduce the heat to low, cover, and simmer for 15-20 minutes or until the lentils and carrots are tender.

6.Stir in the diced tomatoes, including their juice and the coconut milk. Simmer for an additional 5 minutes to heat through and combine the flavors.

7.Using an immersion blender, carefully blend the soup until smooth and creamy. Alternatively, you can transfer the soup in batches to a regular blender and blend until smooth. Be cautious when blending hot liquids.

8.Season the soup with salt and black pepper to taste. Adjust the seasoning as needed.

9.Serve the Curried Lentil and Carrot Soup hot, garnished with fresh cilantro leaves and lime wedges if desired.

NUTRITIONAL FACTS

Calories: 336 kcal Fat: 16g Protein: 11g Carbs: 38g Sugar: 8g Fiber: 11g Vitamin A: 17571 IU (351% DV)

Vitamin C: 13mg (22% DV) Calcium: 60mg (6% DV) Iron: 4mg (22% DV) Potassium: 646mg (18% DV)

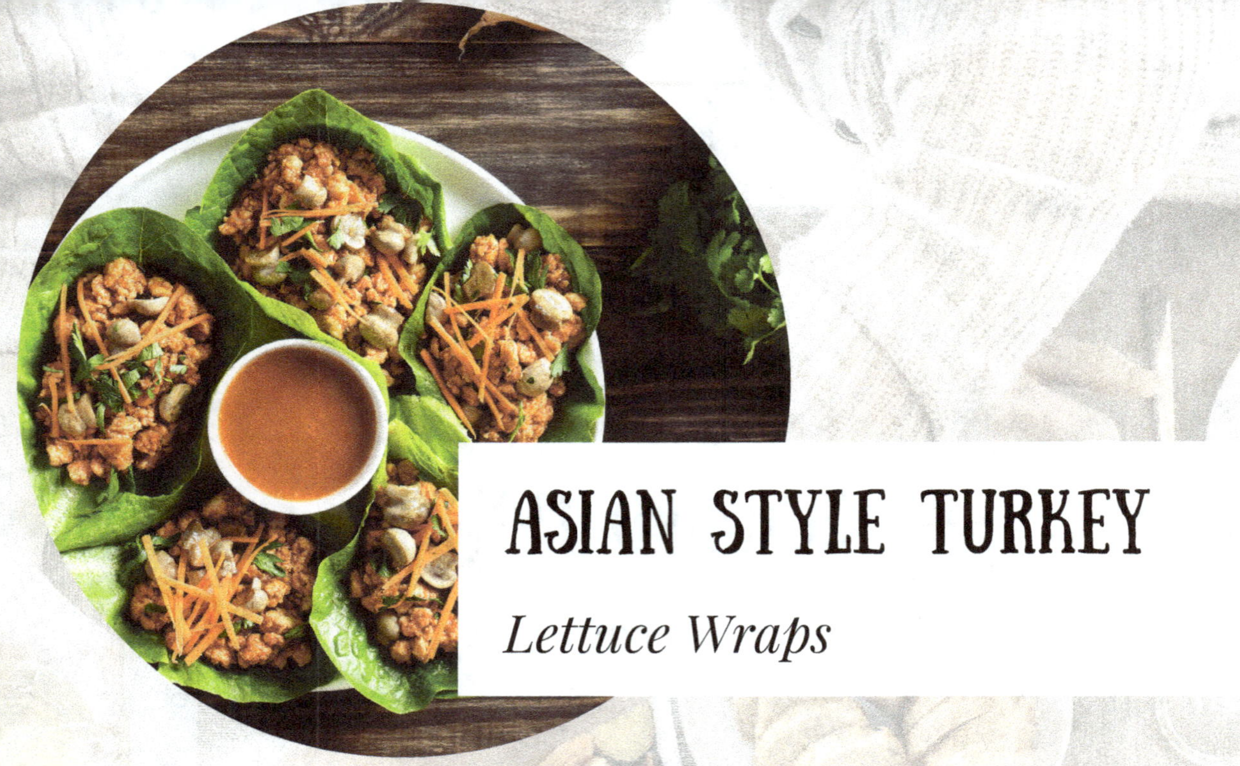

ASIAN STYLE TURKEY

Lettuce Wraps

Prep. Time: 15 minutes | **Cooking Time:** 15 minutes | **Servings:** 4

INGREDIENTS

- ·1 pound lean ground turkey
- ·1 tablespoon sesame oil
- ·1 small onion, finely chopped
- ·2 cloves garlic, minced
- ·1 tablespoon ginger, minced
- ·1/4 cup reduced-sodium soy sauce
- ·2 tablespoons hoisin sauce
- ·1 teaspoon rice vinegar
- ·1 teaspoon sriracha sauce (adjust to taste)
- ·1 cup shiitake mushrooms, finely chopped
- ·1/2 cup water chestnuts, finely chopped
- ·1/4 cup green onions, thinly sliced
- ·1 head of iceberg lettuce, leaves separated, washed and dried
- ·Sesame seeds, for garnish (optional)
- ·Fresh cilantro leaves for garnish (optional)

DIRECTIONS

1. Heat sesame oil in a large skillet or wok over medium-high heat.
2. Add the chopped onion, garlic, and ginger to the skillet. Sauté for 2-3 minutes until the onion becomes translucent and fragrant.
3. Add the ground turkey to the skillet. Break it apart with a spatula until browned and cooked about 5-7 minutes.
4. In a small bowl, mix together the reduced-sodium soy sauce, hoisin sauce, rice vinegar, and sriracha sauce. Stir this sauce mixture into the cooked turkey, coating the meat evenly.
5. Add the chopped shiitake mushrooms and water chestnuts to the skillet. Cook for an additional 2-3 minutes until the mushrooms are tender.
6. Remove the skillet from the heat and stir in the thinly sliced green onions.
7. To serve, spoon the turkey mixture into individual lettuce leaves, creating wraps. Garnish with sesame seeds and fresh cilantro leaves if desired.
8. Enjoy your Asian Style Turkey Lettuce Wraps!

NUTRITIONAL FACTS

Calories: 232 kcal Fat: 10g Protein: 20g Carbs: 14g Sugar: 4g Fiber: 3g Vitamin A: 1658 IU (33% DV) Vitamin C: 4mg (7% DV) Calcium: 34mg (3% DV) Iron: 2mg (12% DV) Potassium: 482mg (14% DV)

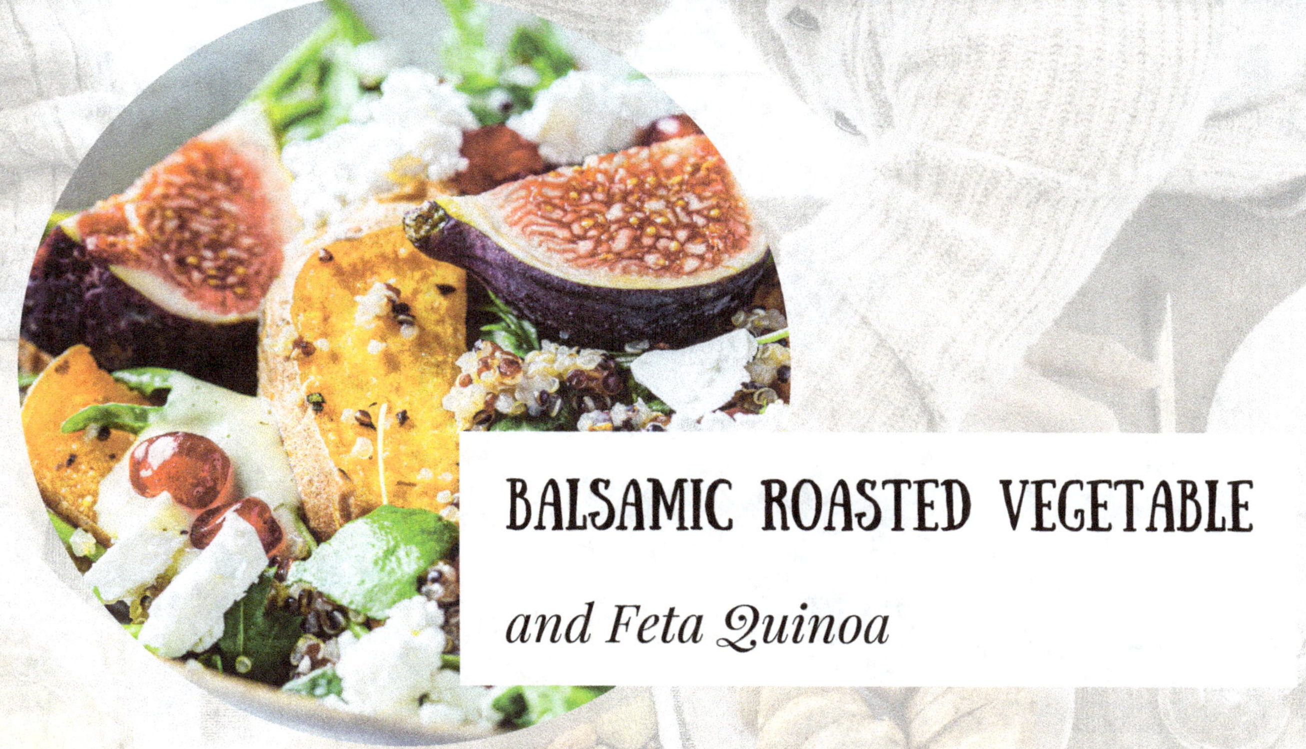

BALSAMIC ROASTED VEGETABLE

and Feta Quinoa

Prep. Time: 15 minutes | **Cooking Time:** 25 minutes | **Servings:** 4

INGREDIENTS

- 1 cup quinoa, rinsed and drained
- 2 cups water
- 2 cups mixed vegetables (e.g., bell peppers, zucchini, cherry tomatoes, red onion), chopped into bite-sized pieces
- 2 tablespoons extra-virgin olive oil
- 2 tablespoons balsamic vinegar
- 1 teaspoon dried oregano
- Salt and pepper to taste
- 1/2 cup crumbled feta cheese
- Fresh basil leaves, for garnish (optional)

DIRECTIONS

1. Preheat your oven to 425°F (220°C).
2. In a medium saucepan, combine the rinsed quinoa and water. Bring to a boil, then reduce the heat to low, cover, and simmer for about 15 minutes or until the quinoa is cooked and the water is absorbed. Remove from heat and let it sit, covered, for 5 minutes. Fluff with a fork and set aside.
3. In a large mixing bowl, combine the chopped mixed vegetables, extra-virgin olive oil, balsamic vinegar, dried oregano, salt, and pepper. Toss to coat the vegetables evenly with the dressing.
4. Spread the coated vegetables in a single layer on a baking sheet lined with parchment paper.
5. Roast the vegetables in the oven for about 20-25 minutes or until they are tender and slightly caramelized, stirring once halfway through cooking.
6. In a serving dish, layer the cooked quinoa, roasted vegetables, and crumbled feta cheese.
7. Garnish with fresh basil leaves if desired.
8. Serve your Balsamic Roasted Vegetable and Feta Quinoa as a hearty and nutritious meal.

NUTRITIONAL FACTS

Calories: 345 kcal Fat: 14g Protein: 10g Carbs: 48g Sugar: 6g Fiber: 6g Vitamin A: 4706 IU (94% DV) Vitamin C: 59mg (98% DV) Calcium: 174mg (17% DV) Iron: 3mg (17% DV) Potassium: 596mg (17% DV)

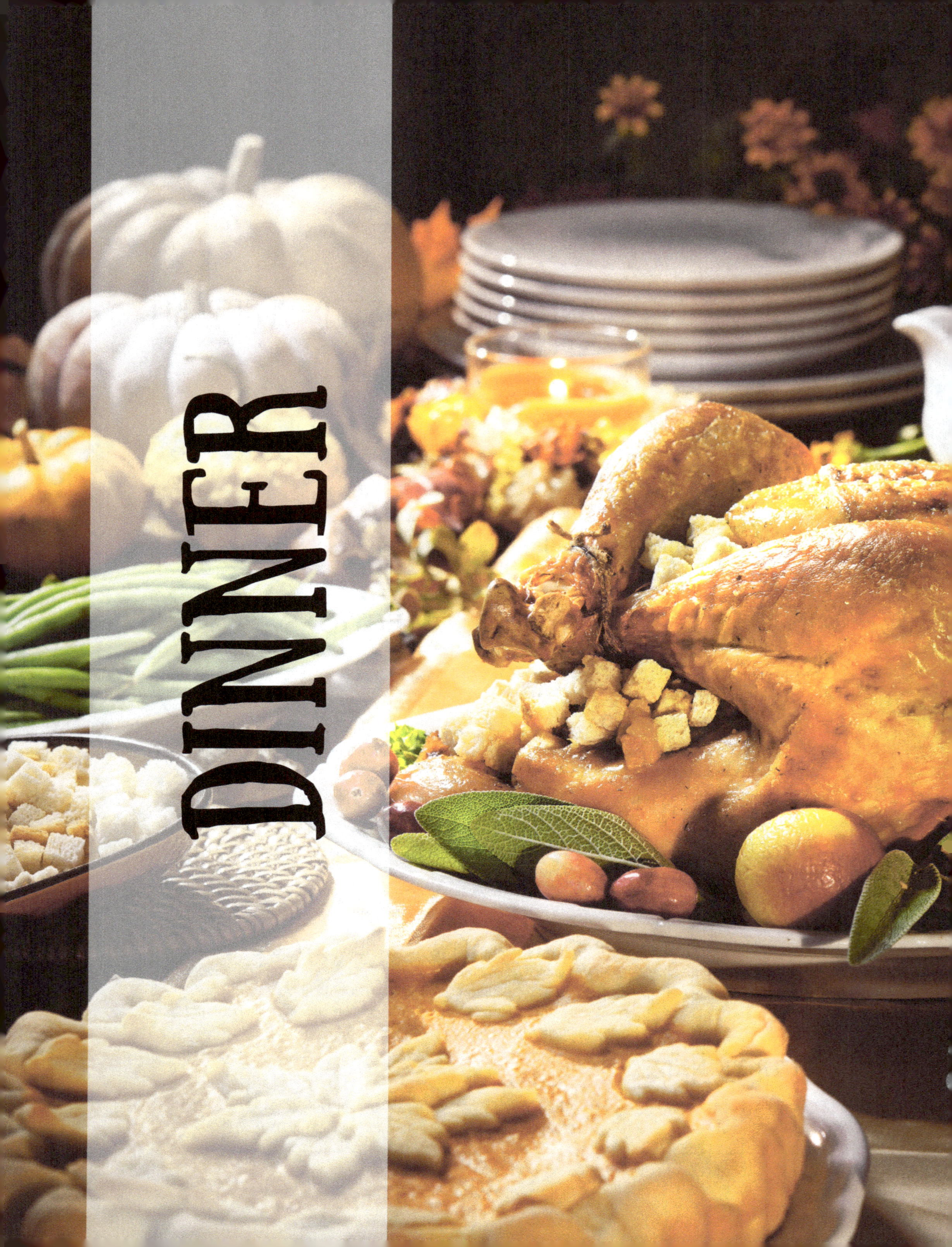
DINNER

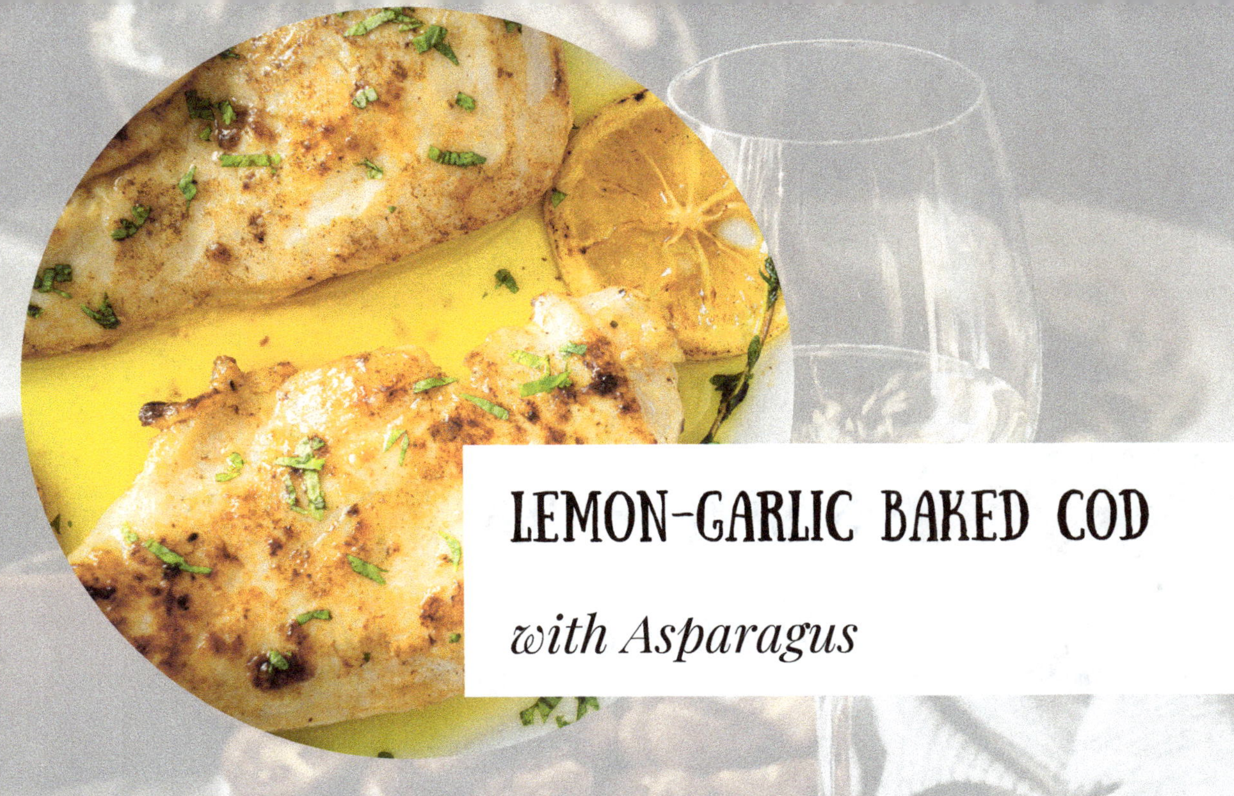

LEMON-GARLIC BAKED COD

with Asparagus

Prep. Time: 10 minutes | **Cooking Time:** 15 minutes | **Servings:** 4

INGREDIENTS

·4 cod fillets (about 6 ounces each)

·1 bunch of fresh asparagus, trimmed

·2 tablespoons olive oil

·3 cloves garlic, minced

·1 lemon, zested and juiced

·2 tablespoons fresh parsley, chopped

·Salt and black pepper to taste

·Lemon slices for garnish (optional)

DIRECTIONS

1. Preheat your oven to 400°F (200°C).
2. Place the trimmed asparagus on a baking sheet, drizzle with 1 tablespoon of olive oil and season with salt and black pepper. Toss to coat evenly.
3. In a small bowl, combine the minced garlic, lemon zest, and chopped fresh parsley.
4. Place the cod fillets on the same baking sheet as the asparagus. Drizzle the remaining 1 tablespoon of olive oil over the cod fillets.
5. Sprinkle the garlic, lemon zest, and parsley mixture evenly over the cod fillets.
6. Squeeze fresh lemon juice over the cod fillets and asparagus.
7. Season the cod fillets with salt and black pepper to taste.
8. Bake in the oven for about 12-15 minutes or until the cod is cooked and flakes easily with a fork. The asparagus should be tender yet crisp.
9. Garnish with lemon slices if desired.
10. Serve the Lemon-Garlic Baked Cod with Asparagus as a healthy and satisfying meal that aligns with the Intermittent Fasting for Women Over 50 Diet. Enjoy!

NUTRITIONAL FACTS

Calories: 260 kcal Fat: 10g Protein: 36g Carbs: 7g Sugar: 2g Fiber: 3g Vitamin A: 15% DV Vitamin C: 30% DV Calcium: 6% DV Iron: 12% DV Potassium: 830mg (18% DV)

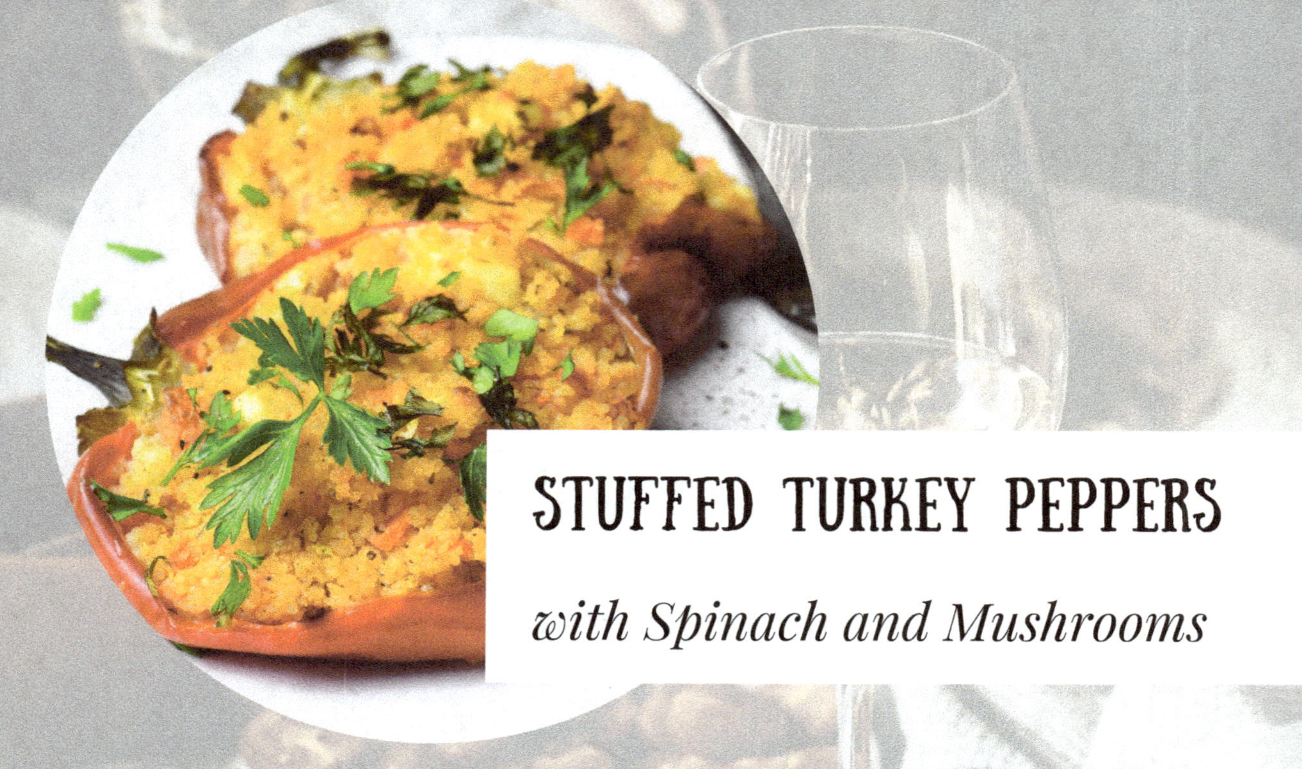

STUFFED TURKEY PEPPERS

with Spinach and Mushrooms

Prep. Time: 20 minutes | **Cooking Time:** 30 minutes | **Servings:** 4

INGREDIENTS

- 4 large bell peppers, any color
- 1 pound ground turkey
- 1 cup mushrooms, finely chopped
- 2 cups fresh spinach, chopped
- 1 small onion, finely chopped
- 2 cloves garlic, minced
- 1 cup cooked quinoa
- 1 cup low-sodium tomato sauce
- 1 teaspoon olive oil
- 1 teaspoon dried oregano
- 1/2 teaspoon dried basil
- Salt and black pepper to taste
- Grated Parmesan cheese for garnish (optional)

DIRECTIONS

1. Preheat your oven to 375°F (190°C).
2. Cut the tops off the bell peppers and remove the seeds and membranes. Set aside.
3. In a large skillet, heat the olive oil over medium heat. Add the chopped onion and garlic, and sauté for 2-3 minutes until they become translucent.
4. Add the ground turkey to the skillet and cook, breaking it apart with a spatula, until it's browned and cooked through about 5 minutes.
5. Stir in the chopped mushrooms, dried oregano, dried basil, salt, and black pepper. Cook for an additional 3-4 minutes until the mushrooms are tender.
6. Add the chopped spinach to the skillet and cook until it wilts about 2 minutes.
7. Stir in the cooked quinoa and 1/2 cup of the tomato sauce. Cook for another 2-3 minutes until everything is well combined. Remove from heat.
8. Stuff each bell pepper with the turkey and vegetable mixture.
9. Place the stuffed peppers in a baking dish and pour the remaining 1/2 cup of tomato sauce over them.
10. Cover the baking dish with foil and bake in the oven for 25-30 minutes or until the peppers are tender.
11. If desired, garnish with grated Parmesan cheese before serving.
12. These Stuffed Turkey Peppers with Spinach and Mushrooms are a balanced and nutritious meal that fits well with the Intermittent Fasting for Women Over 50 Diet. Enjoy!

NUTRITIONAL FACTS

Calories: 330 kcal Fat: 10g Protein: 30g Carbs: 35g Sugar: 8g Fiber: 8g Vitamin A: 130% DV Vitamin C: 270% DV Calcium: 15% DV Iron: 25% DV Potassium: 1150mg (25% DV)

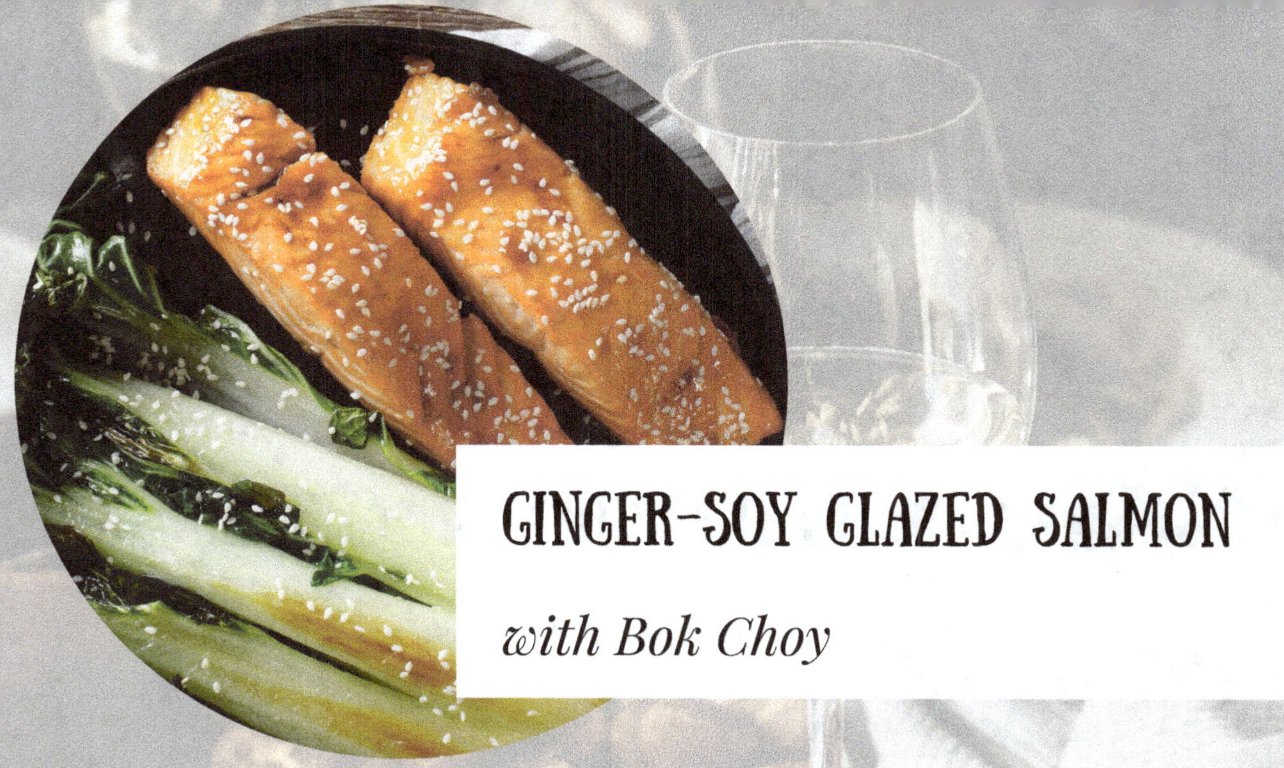

GINGER-SOY GLAZED SALMON

with Bok Choy

Prep. Time: 10 minutes | **Cooking Time:** 15 minutes | **Servings:** 4

INGREDIENTS

- 4 salmon fillets (about 4-6 ounces each)
- 4 baby bok choy heads, halved
- 1/4 cup low-sodium soy sauce
- 2 tablespoons honey
- 1 tablespoon fresh ginger, grated
- 2 cloves garlic, minced
- 1 tablespoon sesame oil
- 1 tablespoon rice vinegar
- 1 teaspoon cornstarch (optional for a thicker glaze)
- Cooking spray or a small amount of oil for cooking
- Sesame seeds and sliced green onions for garnish (optional)

DIRECTIONS

1. In a small bowl, whisk together the soy sauce, honey, grated ginger, minced garlic, sesame oil, and rice vinegar. If you prefer a thicker glaze, add the cornstarch to this mixture. Set aside.
2. Preheat your oven to 375°F (190°C).
3. Heat an oven-safe skillet or pan over medium-high heat and lightly coat it with cooking spray or oil.
4. Place the salmon fillets in the skillet, skin-side down, and sear them for 2-3 minutes until they have a golden-brown crust.
5. Flip the salmon fillets and sear the other side for 2 minutes.
6. Pour the ginger-soy glaze over the salmon fillets in the skillet.
7. Transfer the skillet to the preheated oven and roast for 8-10 minutes or until the salmon is cooked and flakes easily with a fork. The internal temperature of the salmon should reach 145°F (63°C).
8. While the salmon is roasting, steam or blanch the bok choy halves until they are tender but still crisp, about 2-3 minutes. Drain them and set aside.
9. Once the salmon is done, remove it from the oven.
10. Serve the ginger-soy glazed salmon over a bed of steamed bok choy.
11. Garnish with sesame seeds and sliced green onions if desired.
12. This Ginger-Soy Glazed Salmon with Bok Choy is a flavorful and nutritious meal that aligns with the principles of the Intermittent Fasting for Women Over 50 Diet. Enjoy!

NUTRITIONAL FACTS

Calories: 300 kcal Fat: 12g Protein: 34g Carbs: 14g Sugar: 8g Fiber: 2g Vitamin A: 150% DV Vitamin C: 120% DV Calcium: 20% DV Iron: 15% DV Potassium: 800mg (20% DV)

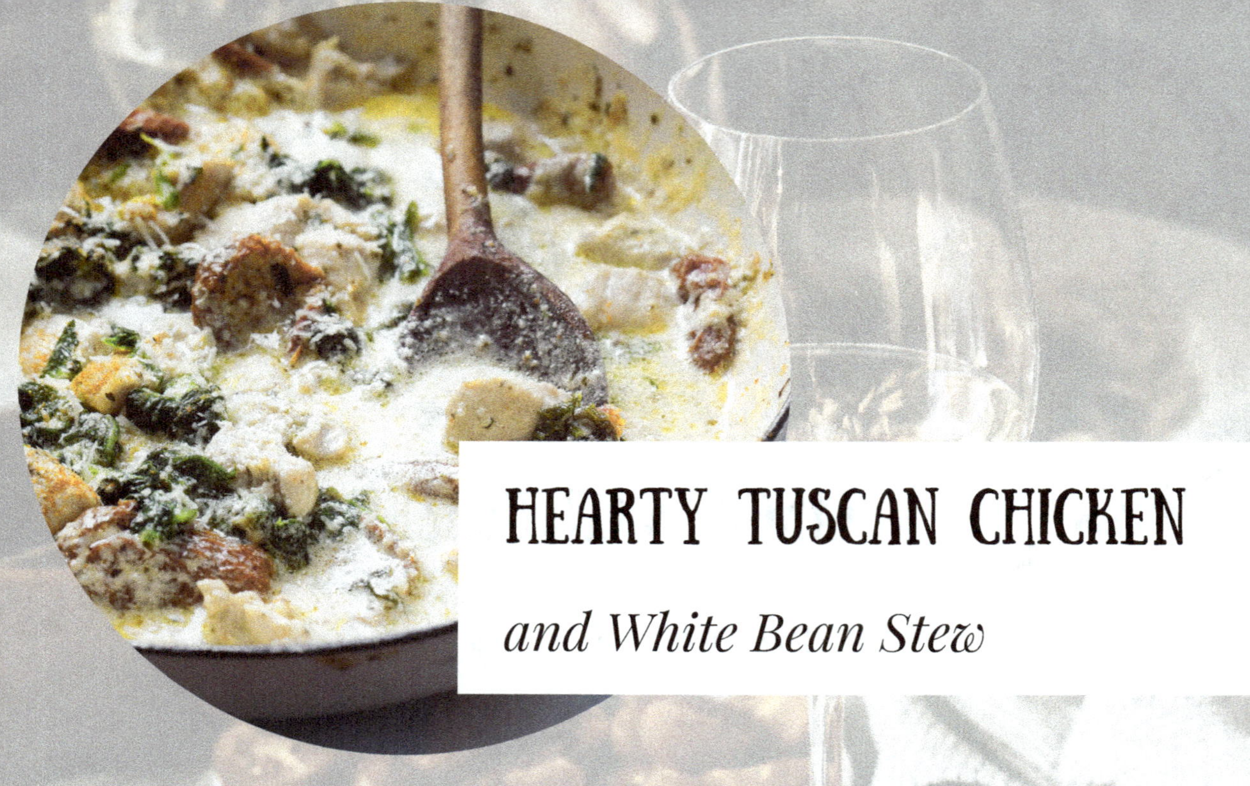

HEARTY TUSCAN CHICKEN

and White Bean Stew

Prep. Time: 15 minutes | **Cooking Time:** 30 minutes | **Servings:** 4

INGREDIENTS

·1 pound boneless, skinless chicken breasts cut into bite-sized pieces

·1 tablespoon olive oil

·1 onion, chopped

·2 cloves garlic, minced

·1 red bell pepper, chopped

·1 yellow bell pepper, chopped

·1 zucchini, diced

·1 can (15 ounces) cannellini beans, drained and rinsed

·1 can (14 ounces) diced tomatoes

·4 cups low-sodium chicken broth

·1 teaspoon dried Italian seasoning

·Salt and black pepper to taste

·2 cups baby spinach leaves

·Fresh basil leaves for garnish (optional)

DIRECTIONS

1. In a large pot or Dutch oven, heat the olive oil over medium heat.

2. Add the chopped onion and cook for 2-3 minutes until it becomes translucent.

3. Stir in the minced garlic and cook for 30 seconds until fragrant.

4. Add the bite-sized chicken pieces to the pot and cook, stirring occasionally, until they are browned on all sides, about 5-7 minutes.

5. Add the chopped red and yellow bell peppers and diced zucchini to the pot. Cook for another 2-3 minutes until the vegetables begin to soften.

6. Pour in the diced tomatoes, cannellini beans, and chicken broth. Stir in the dried Italian seasoning and season with salt and black pepper to taste.

7. Bring the mixture to a boil, then reduce the heat to low and let it simmer for about 20-25 minutes, allowing the flavors to meld together.

8. About 5 minutes before serving, stir in the baby spinach leaves and let them wilt into the stew.

9. Taste and adjust the seasoning if necessary.

10. Serve the Tuscan Chicken and White Bean Stew hot, garnished with fresh basil leaves if desired.

11. This hearty and nutritious stew is an excellent option for those following the Intermittent Fasting for Women Over 50 Diet. Enjoy!

NUTRITIONAL FACTS

Calories: 300 kcal Fat: 6g Protein: 30g Carbs: 30g Sugar: 6g Fiber: 8g Vitamin A: 70% DV Vitamin C: 140% DV Calcium: 10% DV Iron: 25% DV Potassium: 900mg (25% DV)

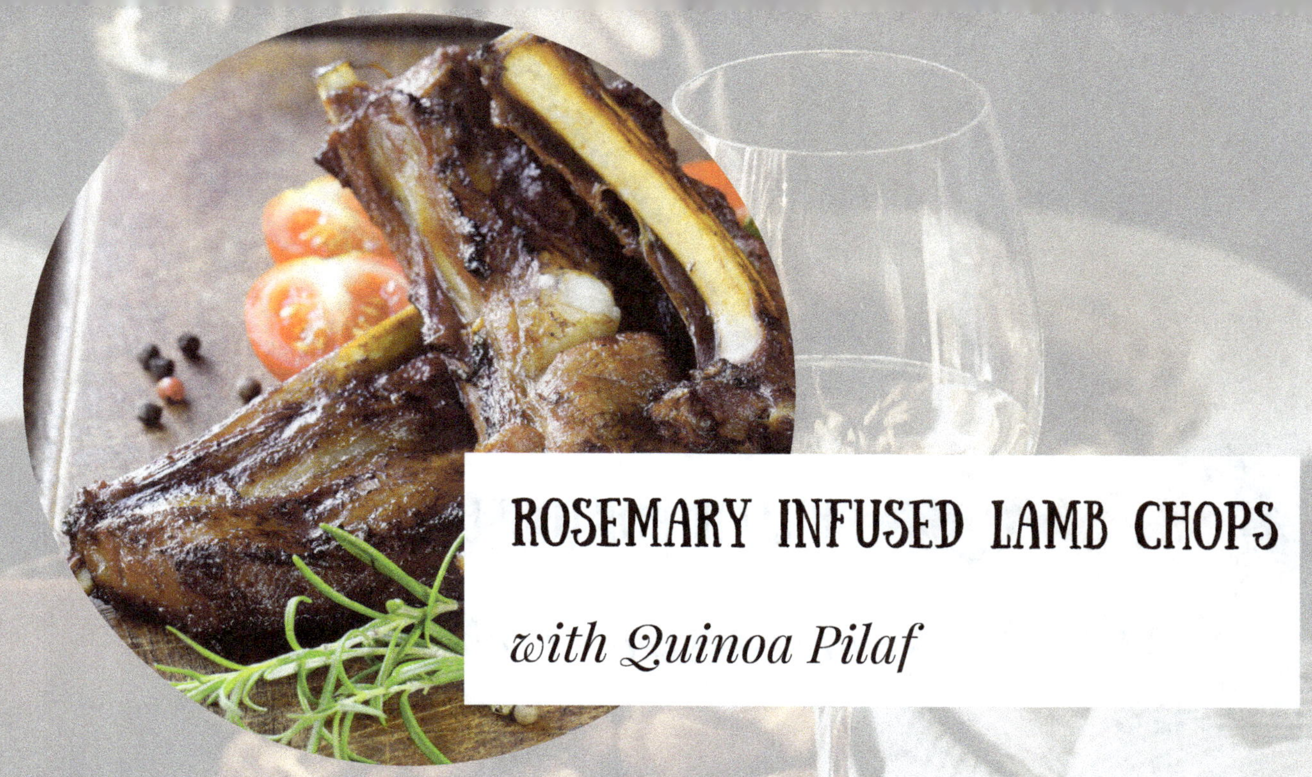

ROSEMARY INFUSED LAMB CHOPS

with Quinoa Pilaf

Prep. Time: 15 minutes | **Cooking Time:** 20 minutes | **Servings:** 4

INGREDIENTS

For Rosemary Infused Lamb Chops:
- 8 lamb loin chops
- 2 tablespoons fresh rosemary leaves, chopped
- 2 cloves garlic, minced
- 2 tablespoons olive oil
- Salt and black pepper to taste

For Quinoa Pilaf:
- 1 cup quinoa, rinsed and drained
- 2 cups low-sodium chicken or vegetable broth
- 1/2 cup diced red bell pepper
- 1/2 cup diced yellow bell pepper
- 1/2 cup diced red onion
- 1/2 cup frozen peas, thawed
- 2 tablespoons olive oil
- 1/4 cup fresh parsley, chopped
- Salt and black pepper to taste

DIRECTIONS

1. In a bowl, combine the chopped rosemary, minced garlic, olive oil, salt, and black pepper. Mix to create a marinade.
2. Place the lamb chops in a resealable plastic bag or a shallow dish. Pour the marinade over the chops, ensuring they are well coated. Seal the bag or cover the dish, and refrigerate for at least 30 minutes to allow the flavors to infuse.
3. Preheat your grill or grill pan to medium-high heat.
4. Remove the lamb chops from the marinade and shake off any excess.
5. Grill the lamb chops for 3-4 minutes per side for medium-rare, or adjust the cooking time to your desired level of doneness.
6. Remove the lamb chops from the grill and let them rest for a few minutes before serving.
7. In a medium saucepan, combine the quinoa and chicken or vegetable broth. Bring to a boil, then reduce the heat to low, cover, and simmer for about 15 minutes until the quinoa is cooked and the liquid is absorbed. Fluff the quinoa with a fork.
8. In a large skillet, heat the olive oil over medium heat. Add the diced red bell pepper, yellow bell pepper, and red onion. Sauté for about 3-4 minutes or until the vegetables are tender.
9. Add the cooked quinoa, thawed peas, chopped parsley, salt, and black pepper to the skillet with the sautéed vegetables. Stir well to combine and heat through for 2-3 minutes.

NUTRITIONAL FACTS

Calories: 470 kcal Fat: 19g Protein: 38g Carbs: 34g Sugar: 3g Fiber: 6g Vitamin A: 25% DV Vitamin C: 80% DV Calcium: 6% DV Iron: 30% DV Potassium: 770mg (20% DV)

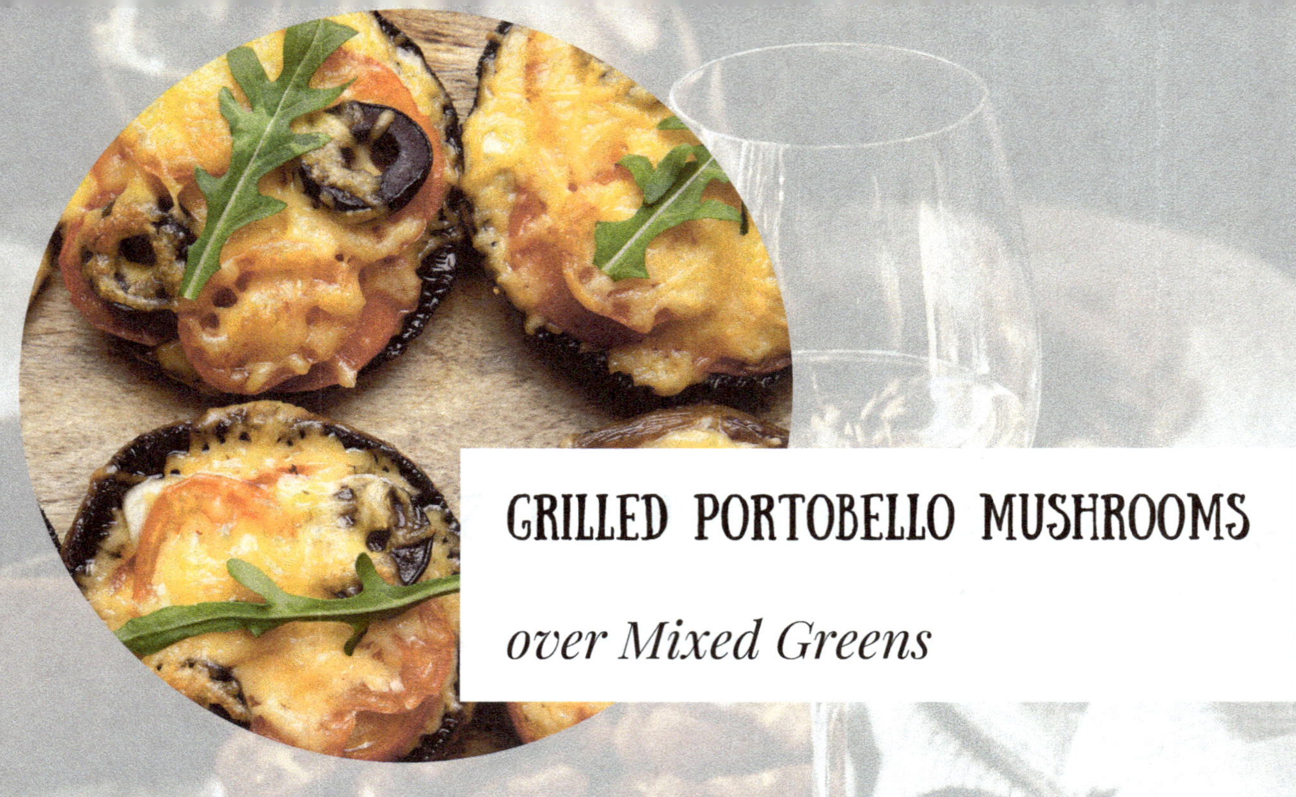

GRILLED PORTOBELLO MUSHROOMS

over Mixed Greens

Prep. Time: 15 minutes | **Cooking Time:** 10 minutes | **Servings:** 4

INGREDIENTS

For Grilled Portobello Mushrooms:
- 4 large Portobello mushrooms, stems removed
- 2 tablespoons balsamic vinegar
- 2 tablespoons olive oil
- 2 cloves garlic, minced
- Salt and black pepper to taste

For Mixed Greens Salad:
- 8 cups mixed salad greens (e.g., arugula, spinach, romaine)
- 1 cup cherry tomatoes, halved
- 1/2 red onion, thinly sliced
- 1/4 cup crumbled feta cheese (optional)
- 2 tablespoons balsamic vinaigrette dressing

DIRECTIONS

1. In a small bowl, whisk together the balsamic vinegar, olive oil, minced garlic, salt, and black pepper to create a marinade.
2. Brush the marinade generously over both sides of the Portobello mushrooms.
3. Preheat your grill or grill pan to medium-high heat.
4. Grill the Portobello mushrooms for 4–5 minutes per side or until they are tender and have grill marks.
5. Remove the grilled mushrooms from the heat and let them rest for a few minutes.
6. In a large salad bowl, combine the mixed salad greens, cherry tomatoes, and thinly sliced red onion.
7. Toss the salad with balsamic vinaigrette dressing until well coated.
8. Place a bed of mixed greens salad on each serving plate.
9. Top the salad with the grilled Portobello mushrooms.
10. Optionally, sprinkle crumbled feta cheese over the mushrooms.

NUTRITIONAL FACTS

Calories: 140 kcal Fat: 9g Protein: 4g Carbs: 13g Sugar: 6g Fiber: 3g Vitamin A: 80% DV Vitamin C: 60% DV

Calcium: 10% DV Iron: 15% DV Potassium: 400mg (10% DV)

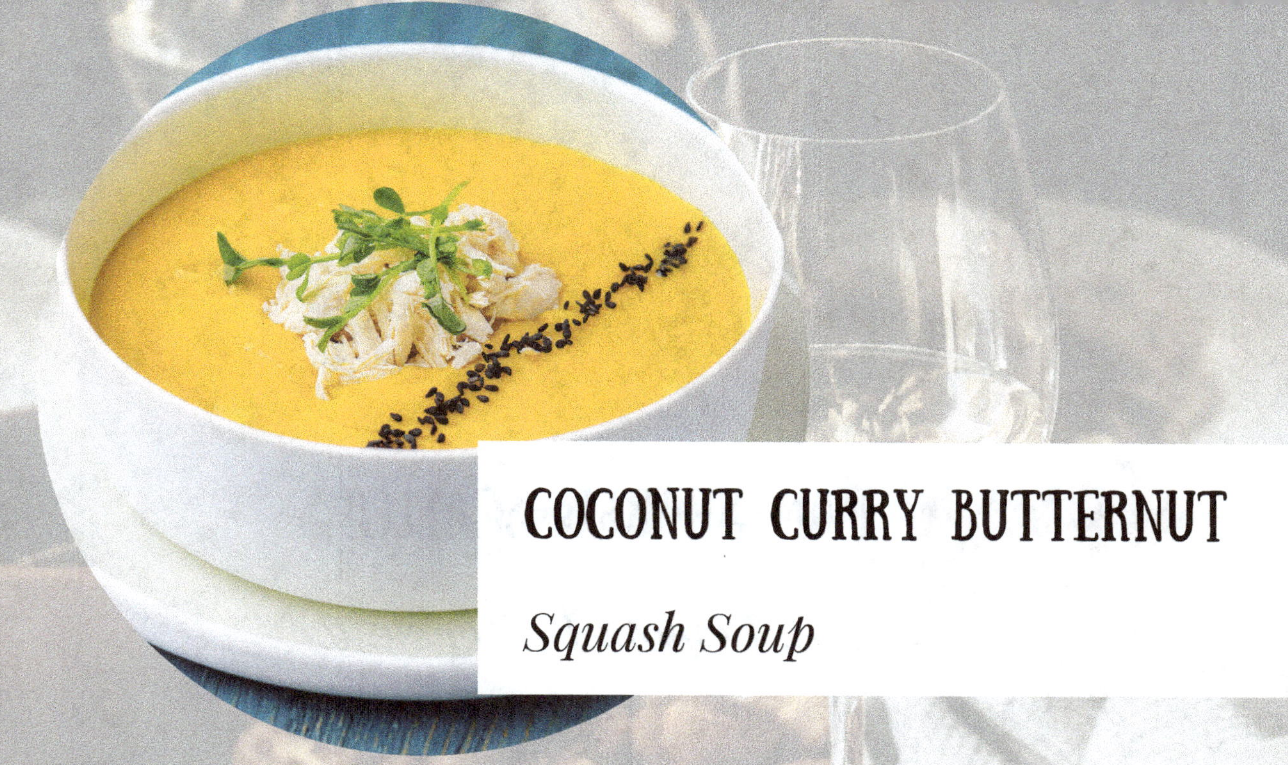

COCONUT CURRY BUTTERNUT

Squash Soup

Prep. Time: 15 minutes | **Cooking Time:** 25 minutes | **Servings:** 4

INGREDIENTS

- 1 medium butternut squash (about 2 pounds), peeled, seeded, and cubed
- 1 can (13.5 oz) unsweetened coconut milk
- 1 onion, chopped
- 2 cloves garlic, minced
- 1 tablespoon fresh ginger, minced
- 1 tablespoon curry powder
- 1/2 teaspoon ground cumin
- 1/2 teaspoon ground coriander
- 1/4 teaspoon cayenne pepper (adjust to taste)
- 4 cups vegetable broth
- 2 tablespoons olive oil
- Salt and black pepper to taste
- Fresh cilantro leaves for garnish (optional)

DIRECTIONS

1. Heat the olive oil in a large pot over medium heat. Add the chopped onion and cook for about 3-4 minutes until it becomes translucent.
2. Stir in the minced garlic and ginger, and cook for 1-2 minutes until fragrant.
3. Add the curry powder, ground cumin, ground coriander, and cayenne pepper to the pot. Cook, stirring constantly, for about 1 minute until the spices are toasted.
4. Add the cubed butternut squash to the pot and season with salt and black pepper. Cook for 5 minutes, stirring occasionally.
5. Pour in the vegetable broth and bring the mixture to a boil. Reduce the heat to low, cover, and simmer for 15-20 minutes or until the butternut squash is tender and easily pierced with a fork.
6. Using an immersion blender or a countertop blender, carefully puree the soup until it's smooth and creamy.
7. Return the soup to the pot (if using a countertop blender) and stir in the coconut milk. Cook for 5 minutes over low heat, allowing the flavors to meld.
8. Taste and adjust the seasoning, adding more salt, black pepper, or cayenne pepper if desired.
9. Serve the Coconut Curry Butternut Squash Soup hot, garnished with fresh cilantro leaves if preferred.

NUTRITIONAL FACTS

Calories: 270 kcal Fat: 21g Protein: 3g Carbs: 22g Sugar: 4g Fiber: 4g Vitamin A: 400% DV Vitamin C: 60% DV Calcium: 10% DV Iron: 10% DV Potassium: 700mg (20% DV)

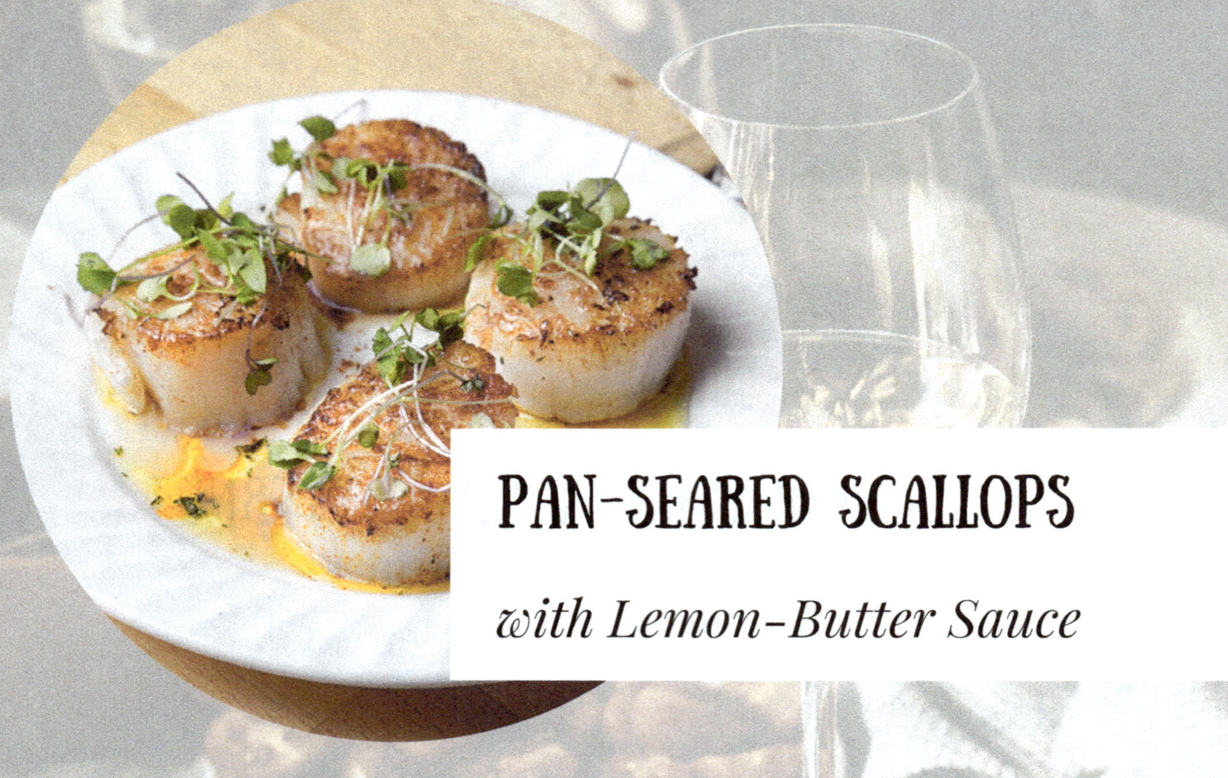

PAN-SEARED SCALLOPS

with Lemon-Butter Sauce

Prep. Time: 10 minutes | **Cooking Time:** 5 minutes | **Servings:** 4

INGREDIENTS

- 1 pound large sea scallops
- 2 tablespoons unsalted butter
- 2 tablespoons olive oil
- Salt and black pepper to taste
- 2 cloves garlic, minced
- Juice of 1 lemon
- Zest of 1 lemon
- 2 tablespoons fresh parsley, chopped
- Lemon wedges for garnish

DIRECTIONS

1. Pat the scallops dry with a paper towel to remove excess moisture. Season both sides of the scallops with salt and black pepper.
2. In a large skillet, heat the olive oil over medium-high heat until it starts to shimmer.
3. Carefully add the scallops to the hot skillet, making sure not to overcrowd them. Leave some space between each scallop to allow for even cooking.
4. Sear the scallops for 2-3 minutes on each side or until they develop a golden-brown crust and are opaque in the center. Avoid overcooking to keep them tender.
5. Remove the scallops from the skillet and transfer them to a plate. Cover them loosely with foil to keep them warm.
6. In the same skillet, add the minced garlic and cook for about 30 seconds until fragrant.
7. Add the unsalted butter to the skillet and let it melt, stirring occasionally.
8. Once the butter is melted, squeeze in the lemon juice and add the lemon zest. Stir to combine.
9. Return the seared scallops to the skillet, coating them with the lemon-butter sauce. Cook for another minute, gently tossing the scallops to coat them evenly with the sauce.
10. Sprinkle fresh chopped parsley over the scallops for added flavor and garnish.
11. Serve the pan-eared scallops with Lemon-Butter Sauce immediately, garnished with lemon wedges.

NUTRITIONAL FACTS

Calories: 250 kcal Fat: 16g Protein: 20g Carbs: 4g Sugar: 0g Fiber: 0g Vitamin C: 10% DV Calcium: 2% DV Iron: 4% DV Potassium: 300mg (8% DV)

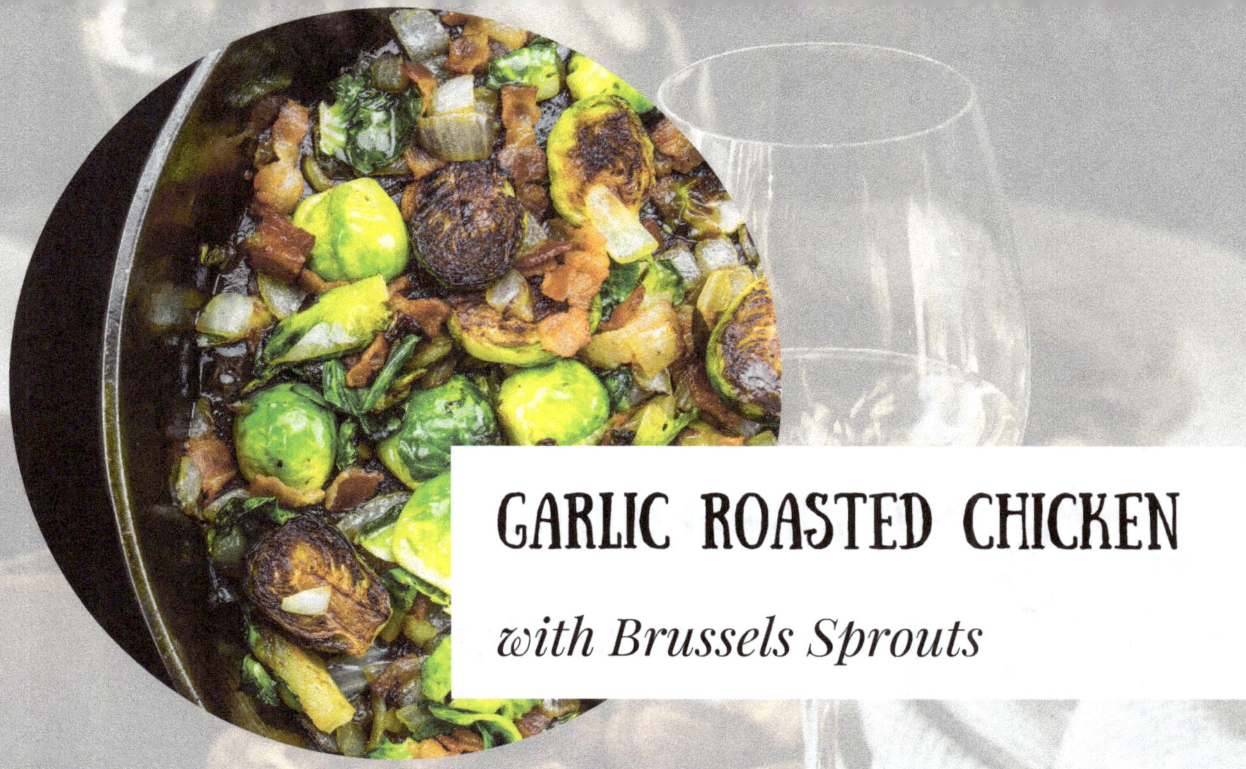

GARLIC ROASTED CHICKEN

with Brussels Sprouts

Prep. Time: 15 minutes | **Cooking Time:** 35 minutes | **Servings:** 4

INGREDIENTS

- 4 bone-in, skin-on chicken thighs
- 1 pound Brussels sprouts, trimmed and halved
- 4 cloves garlic, minced
- 2 tablespoons olive oil
- 1 teaspoon dried thyme
- 1 teaspoon dried rosemary
- Salt and black pepper to taste
- Lemon wedges for garnish (optional)

DIRECTIONS

1. Preheat your oven to 425°F (220°C).
2. In a large bowl, combine the Brussels sprouts, minced garlic, olive oil, dried thyme, dried rosemary, salt, and black pepper. Toss to coat the Brussels sprouts evenly with the seasoning mixture.
3. Season the chicken thighs with salt and black pepper.
4. Heat an oven-safe skillet over medium-high heat. Once hot, add the chicken thighs skin-side down and cook for about 5-7 minutes or until the skin becomes golden brown and crispy. Flip the chicken thighs and cook for an additional 2 minutes.
5. Remove the chicken thighs from the skillet and set them aside.
6. In the same skillet, add the seasoned Brussels sprouts and garlic mixture. Sauté for about 5 minutes, stirring occasionally, until the Brussels sprouts start to brown.
7. Place the seared chicken thighs on top of the Brussels sprouts in the skillet.
8. Transfer the skillet to the preheated oven and roast for about 20-25 minutes, or until the chicken reaches an internal temperature of 165°F (74°C) and the Brussels sprouts are tender.
9. Optional: If desired, broil for 2-3 minutes to crisp up the chicken skin.
10. Garnish with lemon wedges if you like before serving.
11. Divide the Garlic Roasted Chicken with Brussels Sprouts among four plates. Enjoy this flavorful and satisfying dish that fits well within the Intermittent Fasting for Women Over 50 Diet.

NUTRITIONAL FACTS

Calories: 390 kcal Fat: 25g Protein: 27g Carbs: 15g Sugar: 3g Fiber: 6g Vitamin C: 130% DV Calcium: 8% DV Iron: 15% DV Potassium: 750mg (16% DV)

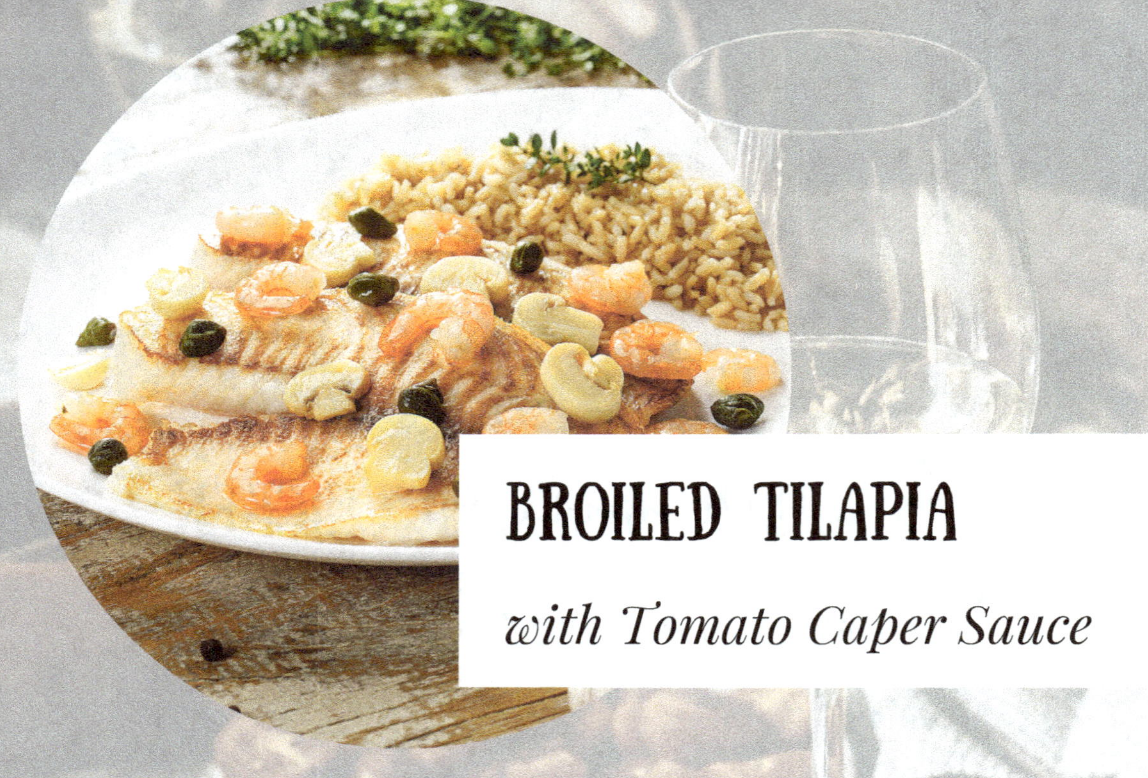

BROILED TILAPIA

with Tomato Caper Sauce

Prep. Time: 10 minutes | **Cooking Time:** 15 minutes | **Servings:** 4

INGREDIENTS

For the Broiled Tilapia:
- 4 tilapia fillets (about 6 ounces each)
- 2 tablespoons olive oil
- Salt and black pepper to taste
- 1 lemon, sliced (for garnish)

For the Tomato Caper Sauce:
- 1 can (14.5 ounces) diced tomatoes, drained
- 2 cloves garlic, minced
- 2 tablespoons capers, drained and rinsed
- 1 tablespoon olive oil
- 1 teaspoon dried basil
- 1/2 teaspoon dried oregano
- Salt and black pepper to taste

DIRECTIONS

1. Position the oven rack about 6 inches below the broiler element and preheat your oven's broiler.
2. Place the tilapia fillets on a baking sheet lined with aluminum foil.
3. Brush both sides of the fillets with olive oil and season with salt and black pepper.
4. Place the baking sheet with the tilapia fillets under the broiler.
5. Broil 6-8 minutes on each side or until the tilapia is opaque and flakes easily with a fork. The exact cooking time may vary based on the thickness of the fillets.
6. While the tilapia is broiling, heat 1 tablespoon of olive oil in a saucepan over medium heat.
7. Add the minced garlic and sauté for about 1 minute or until fragrant.
8. Stir in the drained diced tomatoes, capers, dried basil, oregano, salt, and black pepper.
9. Cook the sauce for 5-7 minutes, stirring occasionally, until it thickens slightly.
10. Once the tilapia fillets are done, remove them from the oven.
11. Spoon the tomato caper sauce over the broiled tilapia fillets.
12. Garnish with lemon slices.
13. Serve the Broiled Tilapia with Tomato Caper Sauce hot, accompanied by your choice of side dishes or steamed vegetables.

NUTRITIONAL FACTS

Calories: 240 kcal Fat: 12g Protein: 31g Carbs: 5g Sugar: 2g Fiber: 2g Vitamin C: 15% DV Calcium: 6% DV Iron: 10% DV Potassium: 520mg (11% DV)

VEGETABLES

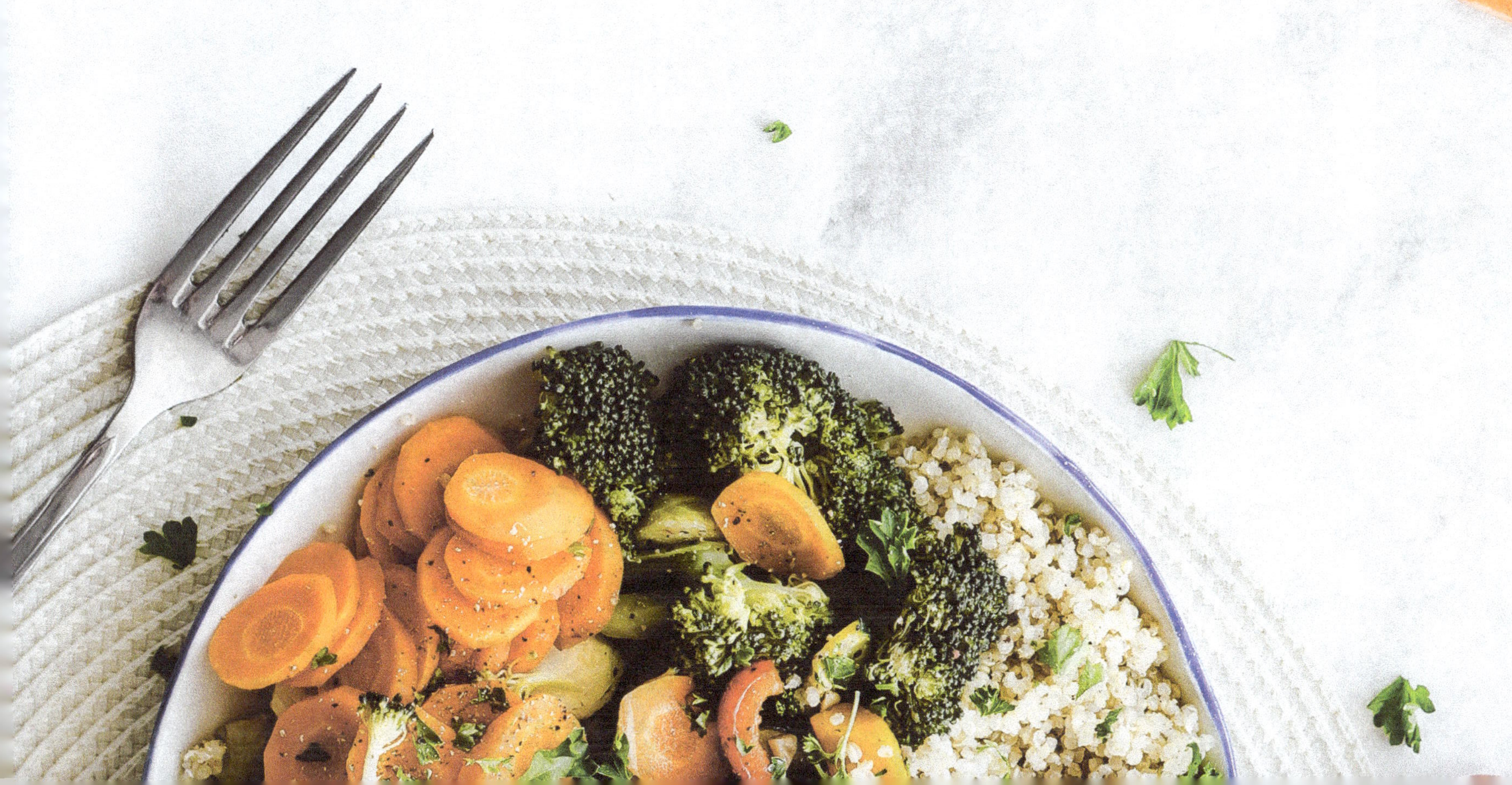

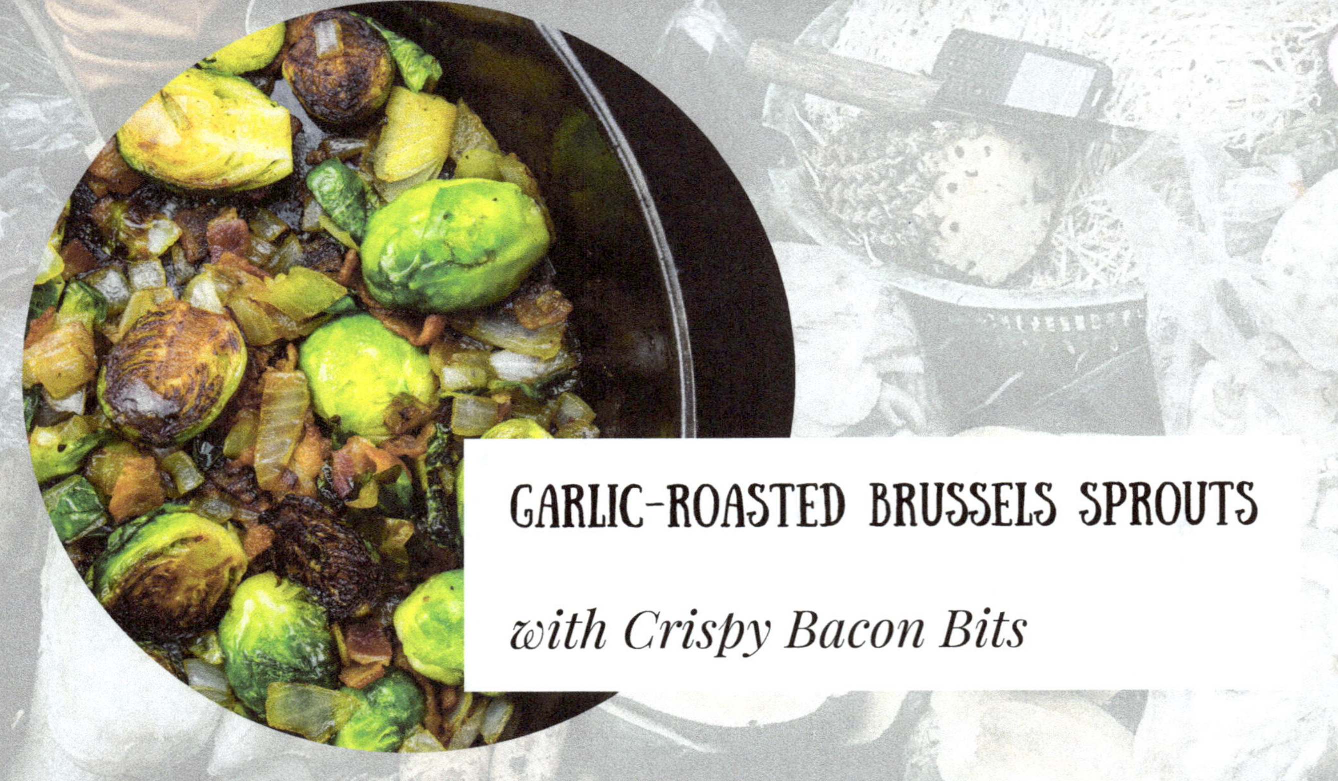

GARLIC-ROASTED BRUSSELS SPROUTS

with Crispy Bacon Bits

Prep. Time: 10 minutes | **Cooking Time:** 25 minutes | **Servings:** 4

INGREDIENTS

·1 pound Brussels sprouts, trimmed and halved

·4 slices of lean bacon, chopped

·2 cloves garlic, minced

·1 tablespoon olive oil

·1/2 teaspoon salt

·1/4 teaspoon black pepper

·1/4 teaspoon red pepper flakes (optional)

·Cooking spray

DIRECTIONS

1. Preheat your oven to 425°F (220°C). Line a baking sheet with aluminum foil and lightly coat it with cooking spray.
2. In a large mixing bowl, combine the trimmed and halved Brussels sprouts, minced garlic, olive oil, salt, black pepper, and red pepper flakes (if using). Toss everything together until the Brussels sprouts are evenly coated with the seasonings.
3. Spread the seasoned Brussels sprouts in a single layer on the prepared baking sheet, ensuring they are not overcrowded. This allows them to roast evenly.
4. In a separate skillet, cook the chopped bacon over medium-high heat until it becomes crispy, about 5-7 minutes. Use a slotted spoon to remove the bacon bits from the skillet and place them on a paper towel-lined plate to drain excess grease.
5. Place the baking sheet with the Brussels sprouts in the preheated oven and roast for 20-25 minutes or until they are tender and have developed a nice golden brown color, stirring once halfway through the cooking time.
6. Remove the roasted Brussels sprouts from the oven and immediately sprinkle the crispy bacon bits over the top.
7. Serve the Garlic-Roasted Brussels Sprouts with Crispy Bacon Bits hot, and enjoy your delicious and satisfying meal!

NUTRITIONAL FACTS

Calories: 180 Fat: 11g Protein: 9g Carbs: 15g Sugar: 3g Fiber: 5g Vitamin A: 20% DV Vitamin C: 160% DV Calcium: 6% DV Iron: 10% DV

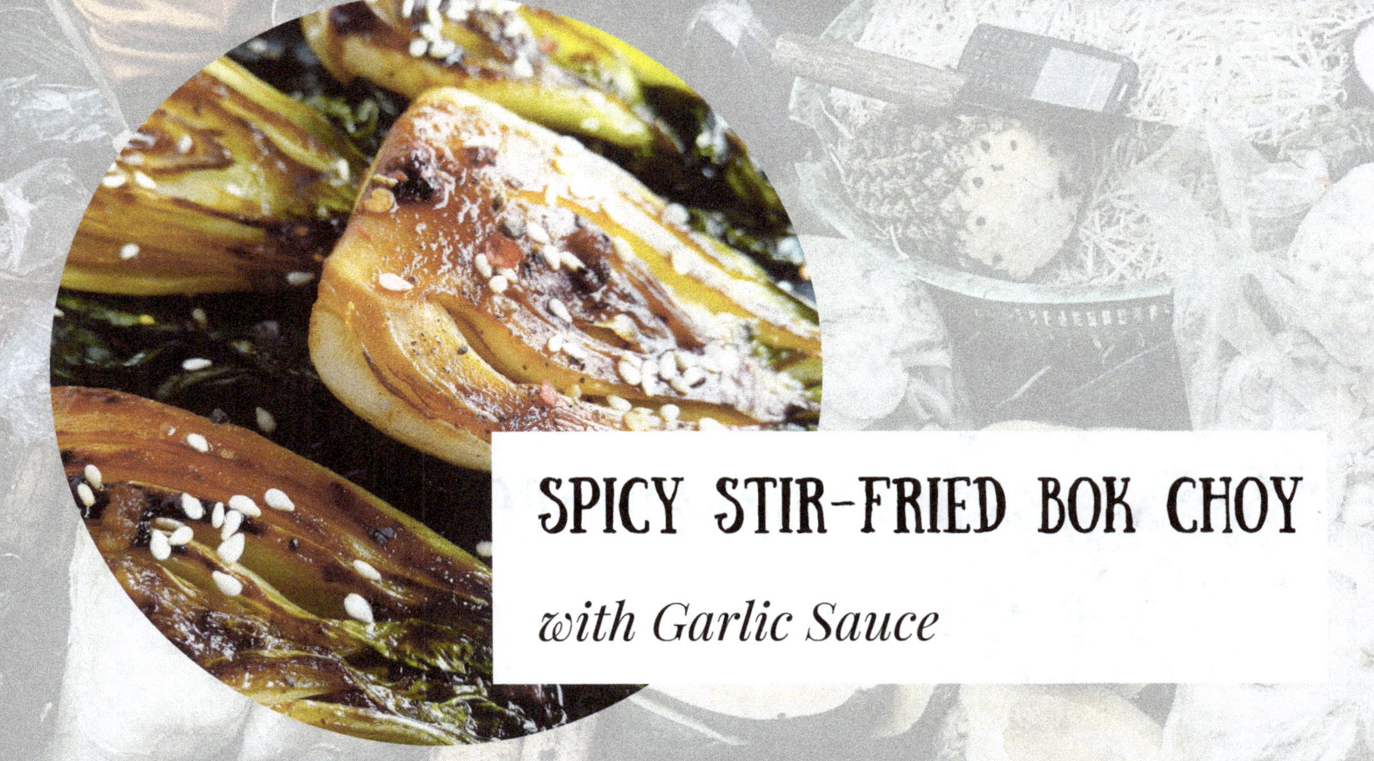

SPICY STIR-FRIED BOK CHOY

with Garlic Sauce

Prep. Time: 10 minutes | **Cooking Time:** 10 minutes | **Servings:** 4

INGREDIENTS

- 1 pound baby bok choy, rinsed and trimmed
- 2 tablespoons low-sodium soy sauce
- 1 tablespoon rice vinegar
- 1 tablespoon sesame oil
- 2 cloves garlic, minced
- 1 teaspoon fresh ginger, minced
- 1/2 teaspoon red pepper flakes (adjust to taste for spiciness)
- 1 teaspoon cornstarch
- 1 tablespoon water
- 1 tablespoon cooking oil (such as canola or peanut oil)
- Optional garnish: toasted sesame seeds and sliced green onions

DIRECTIONS

1. In a small bowl, whisk together the low-sodium soy sauce, rice vinegar, sesame oil, minced garlic, minced ginger, and red pepper flakes. Set this garlic sauce aside.
2. In another small bowl, mix the cornstarch and water to create a slurry. This will be used to thicken the sauce later.
3. Heat a large wok or skillet over high heat. Add the cooking oil and swirl it to coat the pan evenly.
4. Add the baby bok choy to the hot wok or skillet. Stir-fry the bok choy for about 2-3 minutes or until it begins to wilt and the stems become tender.
5. Pour the garlic sauce over the stir-fried bok choy and toss to combine. Allow it to cook for 1-2 minutes, allowing the flavors to meld and the sauce to slightly thicken.
6. Drizzle the cornstarch slurry over the bok choy and stir-fry for another 1-2 minutes until the sauce thickens and coats the bok choy evenly.
7. Remove the spicy stir-fried bok choy from the heat and transfer it to a serving dish.
8. Garnish with toasted sesame seeds and sliced green onions, if desired.
9. Serve the Spicy Stir-Fried Bok Choy with Garlic Sauce hot as a delicious and nutritious side dish or over a bed of brown rice for a complete meal.

NUTRITIONAL FACTS

Calories: 70 Fat: 5g Protein: 2g Carbs: 5g Sugar: 1g Fiber: 2g Vitamin A: 90% DV Vitamin C: 70% DV

Calcium: 10% DV Iron: 6% DV

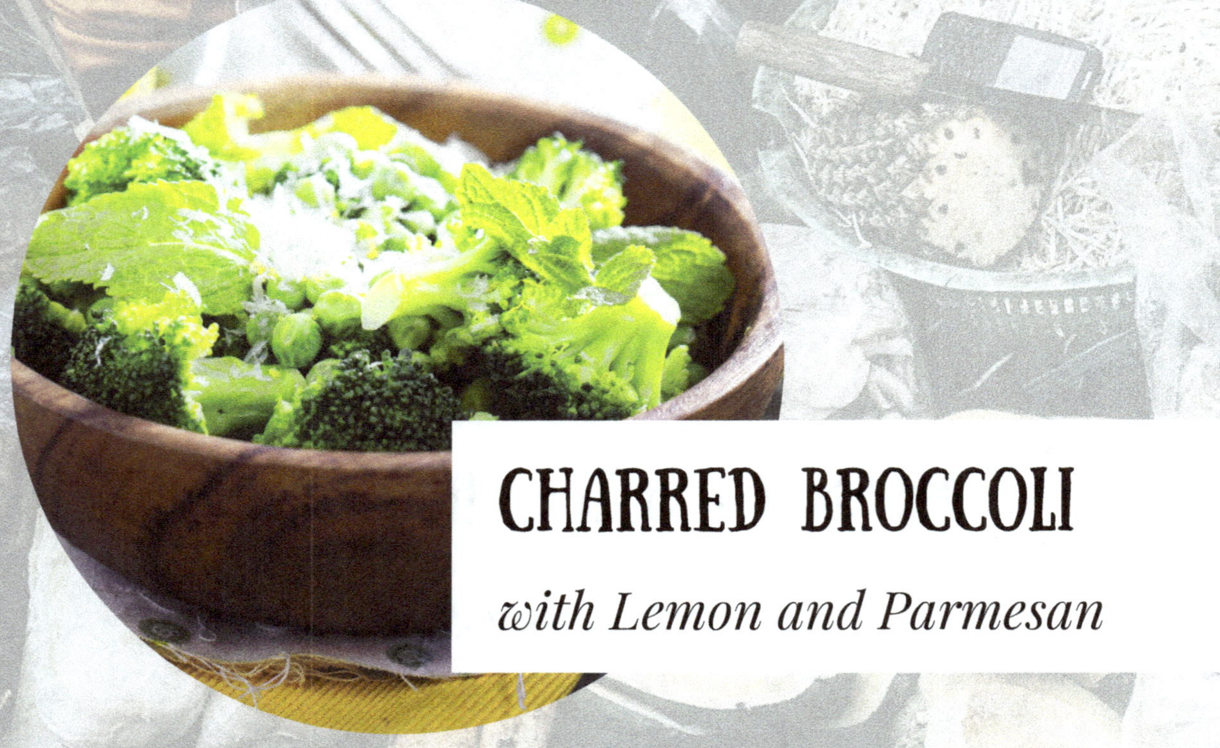

CHARRED BROCCOLI

with Lemon and Parmesan

Prep. Time: 10 minutes | **Cooking Time:** 15 minutes | **Servings:** 4

INGREDIENTS

·1 pound fresh broccoli florets
·2 tablespoons olive oil
·2 cloves garlic, minced
·Zest of 1 lemon
·Juice of 1 lemon
·2 tablespoons grated
Parmesan cheese
·Salt and pepper to taste
·Lemon wedges for garnish
(optional)

DIRECTIONS

1. Preheat your oven to 425°F (220°C). Line a baking sheet with aluminum foil or parchment paper.
2. In a large mixing bowl, toss the broccoli florets with olive oil, minced garlic, lemon zest, salt, and pepper. Ensure that the broccoli is evenly coated with the oil and seasonings.
3. Spread the seasoned broccoli in a single layer on the prepared baking sheet.
4. Roast the broccoli in the oven for 12-15 minutes or until it becomes tender and slightly charred at the edges. Make sure to stir or shake the baking sheet halfway through the cooking time for even char and cooking.
5. Once the broccoli is roasted to your desired char level, remove it from the oven.
6. Drizzle the lemon juice over the charred broccoli and sprinkle the grated Parmesan cheese.
7. Gently toss the broccoli to distribute the lemon juice and Parmesan cheese evenly.
8. Transfer the Charred Broccoli with Lemon and Parmesan to a serving platter.
9. Garnish with lemon wedges if desired.
10. Serve hot as a flavorful and nutritious side dish or light meal.

NUTRITIONAL FACTS

Calories: 100 Fat: 7g Protein: 4g Carbs: 8g Sugar: 2g Fiber: 3g Vitamin A: 20% DV
Vitamin C: 160% DV Calcium: 10% DV Iron: 6% DV

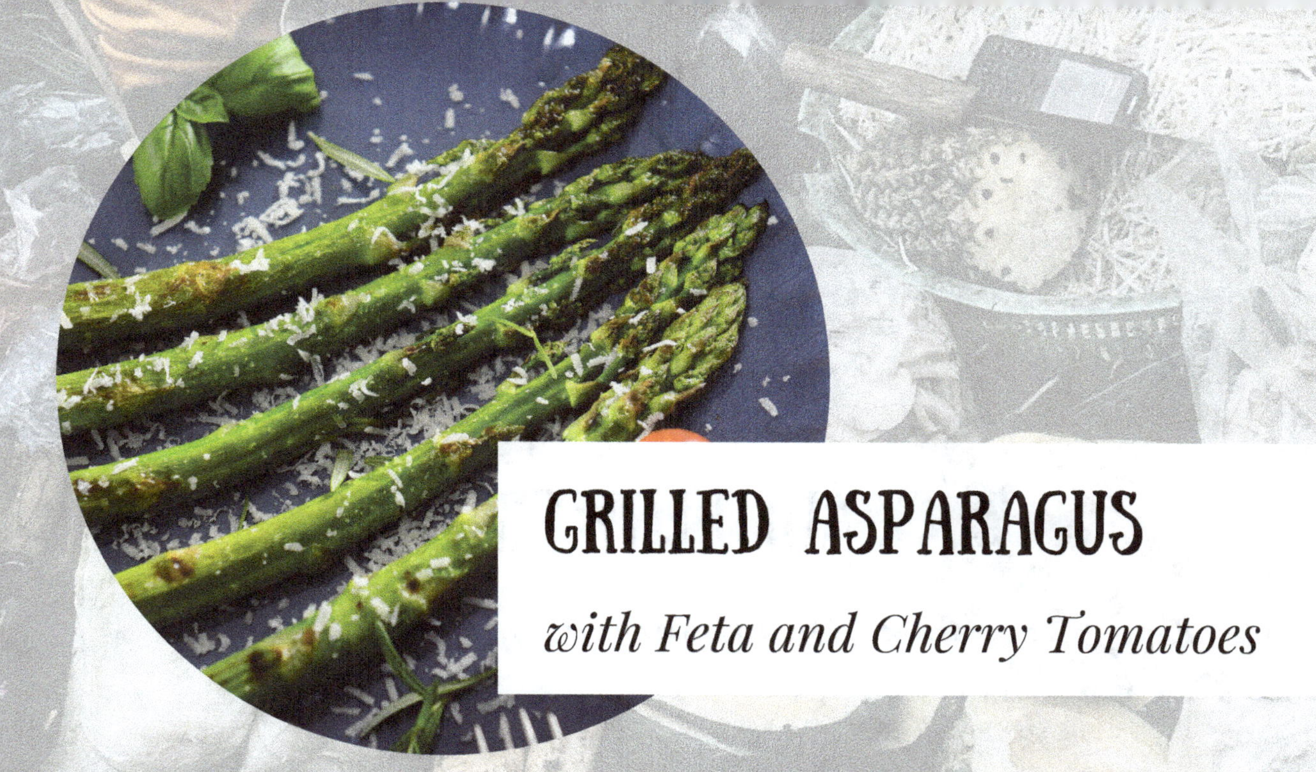

GRILLED ASPARAGUS

with Feta and Cherry Tomatoes

Prep. Time: 10 minutes | **Cooking Time:** 10 minutes | **Servings:** 4

INGREDIENTS

- 1 pound fresh asparagus spears, tough ends trimmed
- 1 cup cherry tomatoes, halved
- 2 tablespoons olive oil
- 2 cloves garlic, minced
- 1/4 cup crumbled feta cheese
- Salt and pepper to taste
- Fresh basil leaves for garnish (optional)

DIRECTIONS

1. Preheat your grill to medium-high heat.
2. In a large mixing bowl, toss the trimmed asparagus spears with olive oil, minced garlic, salt, and pepper. Make sure the asparagus is evenly coated.
3. Thread the asparagus onto grill skewers or use a grill basket to prevent them from falling through the grates.
4. Place the asparagus skewers or grill basket on the preheated grill and cook for about 5-7 minutes, turning occasionally, until the asparagus becomes tender and slightly charred.
5. While the asparagus grills, halve the cherry tomatoes and crumble the feta cheese.
6. Remove the grilled asparagus and transfer them to a serving platter.
7. Sprinkle the halved cherry tomatoes and crumbled feta cheese over the grilled asparagus.
8. Garnish with fresh basil leaves if desired.
9. Serve the Grilled Asparagus with Feta and Cherry Tomatoes hot as a delightful and nutritious side dish.

NUTRITIONAL FACTS

Calories: 110 Fat: 8g Protein: 5g Carbs: 7g Sugar: 3g Fiber: 3g Vitamin A: 20% DV Vitamin C: 35% DV Calcium: 10% DV Iron: 6% DV

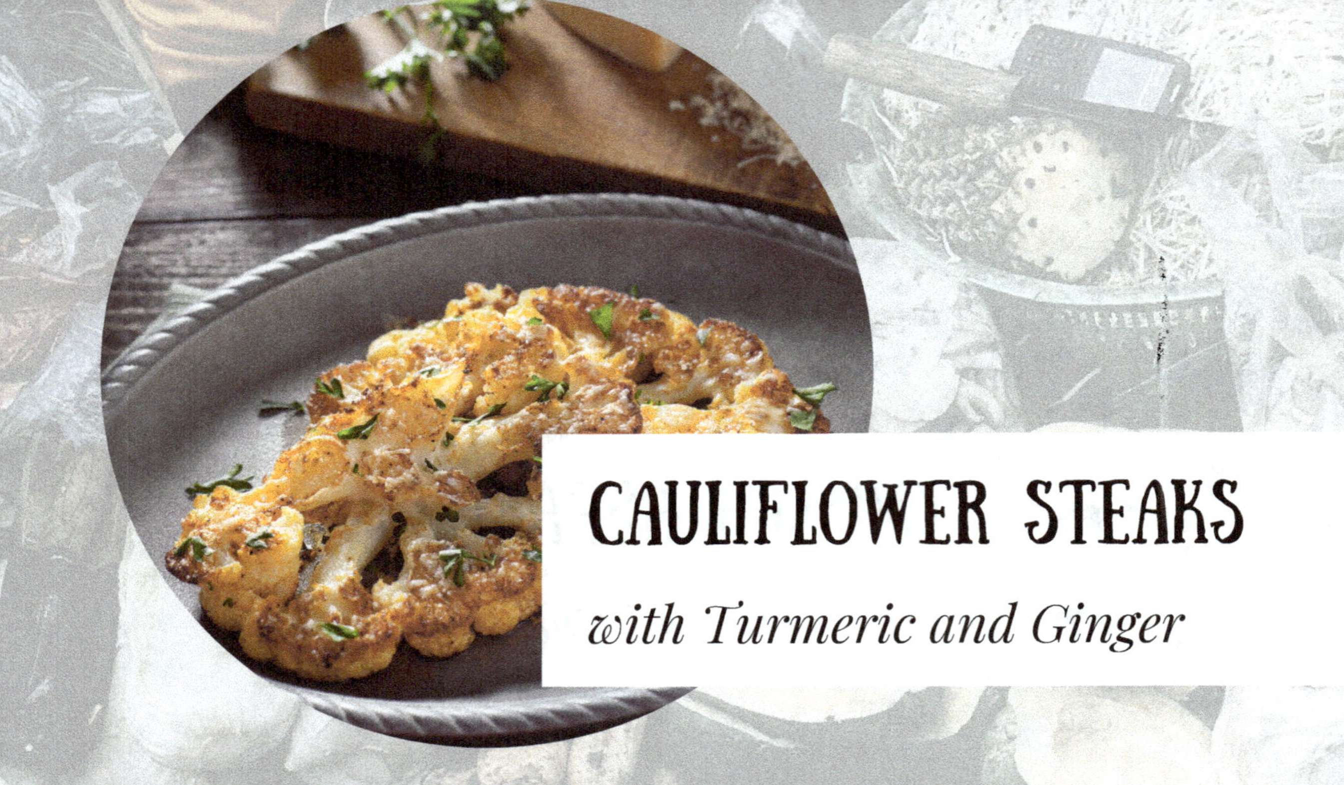

CAULIFLOWER STEAKS

with Turmeric and Ginger

Prep. Time: 10 minutes | **Cooking Time:** 20 minutes | **Servings:** 4

INGREDIENTS

- 1 large head of cauliflower
- 2 tablespoons olive oil
- 1 teaspoon ground turmeric
- 1 teaspoon ground ginger
- Salt and pepper to taste
- Fresh parsley or cilantro for garnish (optional)

DIRECTIONS

1. Preheat your oven to 425°F (220°C). Line a baking sheet with parchment paper.
2. Remove the outer leaves from the cauliflower and trim the stem to create a flat base. Carefully slice the cauliflower into 4 thick "steaks," each about 1-inch (2.5 cm) wide. Reserve any smaller florets that may fall off for later use.
3. In a small bowl, combine the olive oil, ground turmeric, ground ginger, salt, and pepper to create a spice mixture.
4. Place the cauliflower steaks on the prepared baking sheet, ensuring they are evenly spaced.
5. Brush both sides of each cauliflower steak with the spice mixture, ensuring they are well coated.
6. Roast the cauliflower steaks in the preheated oven for about 15-20 minutes, or until they are tender and lightly browned, flipping them halfway through the cooking time.
7. While the cauliflower steaks roast, you can steam or sauté the reserved cauliflower florets as a side dish.
8. Remove the cauliflower steaks from the oven and transfer them to a serving platter.
9. Garnish with fresh parsley or cilantro, if desired.
10. Serve the Cauliflower Steaks with Turmeric and Ginger hot as a flavorful and satisfying main course or side dish.

NUTRITIONAL FACTS

Calories: 90 Fat: 7g Protein: 3g Carbs: 7g Sugar: 3g Fiber: 3g Vitamin A: 0% DV Vitamin C: 130% DV Calcium: 4% DV Iron: 6% DV

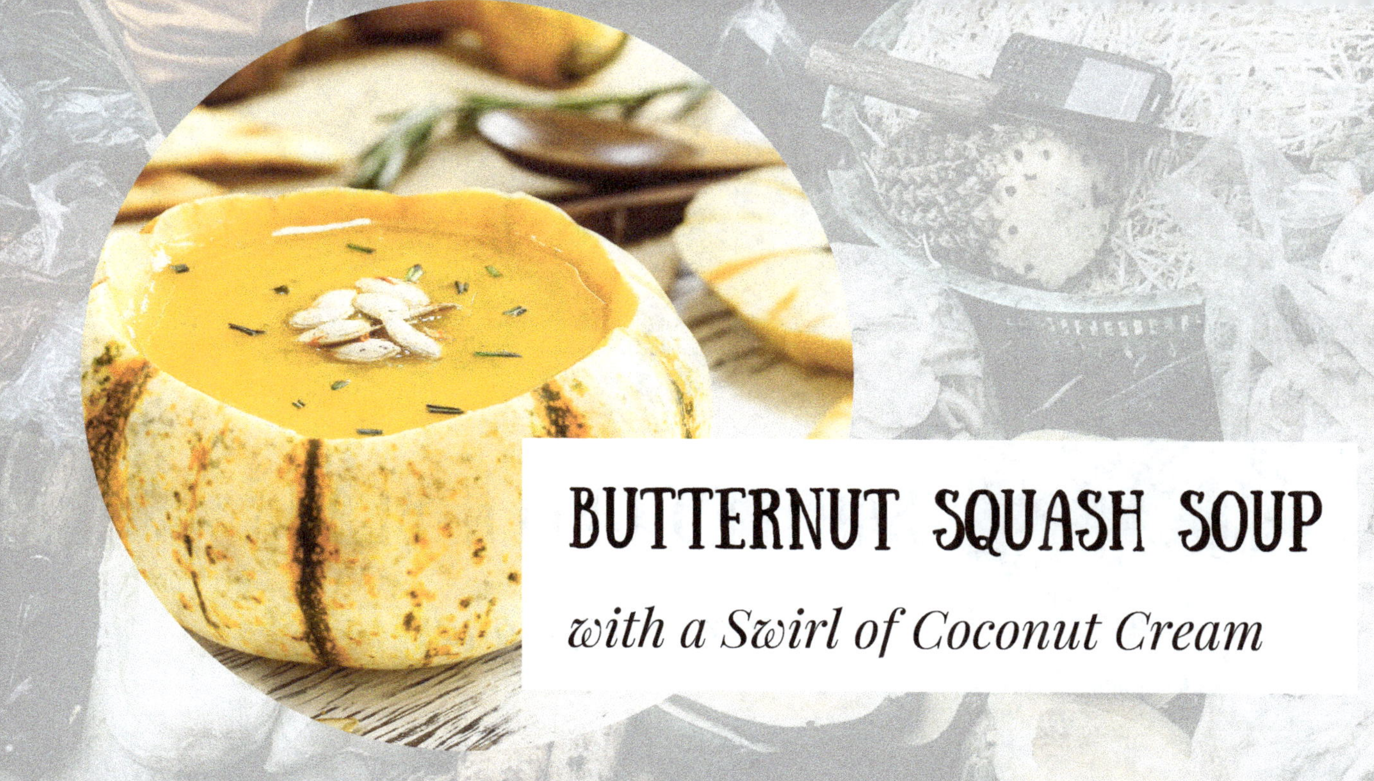

BUTTERNUT SQUASH SOUP

with a Swirl of Coconut Cream

Prep. Time: 15 minutes | **Cooking Time:** 30 minutes | **Servings:** 6

INGREDIENTS

·1 medium butternut squash (about 2 pounds), peeled, seeded, and cubed
·1 large onion, chopped
·2 cloves garlic, minced
·1 tablespoon olive oil
·4 cups low-sodium vegetable broth
·1 teaspoon ground cinnamon
·1/2 teaspoon ground nutmeg
·Salt and pepper to taste
·1/2 cup light coconut milk
·Fresh chives or parsley for garnish (optional)

DIRECTIONS

1. In a large soup pot or Dutch oven, heat the olive oil over medium heat. Add the chopped onion and garlic, and sauté for 2-3 minutes until they become fragrant and translucent.
2. Add the cubed butternut squash to the pot and sauté for another 5 minutes, allowing it to slightly brown.
3. Pour the low-sodium vegetable broth, ground cinnamon, ground nutmeg, salt, and pepper. Stir to combine.
4. Bring the mixture to a boil, reduce the heat to low, cover the pot, and simmer for about 20-25 minutes, or until the butternut squash is tender and easily pierced with a fork.
5. Using an immersion blender, puree the soup until smooth and creamy. Alternatively, you can carefully transfer the soup in batches to a blender and blend until smooth, then return it to the pot.
6. Stir in the light coconut milk, which adds creaminess and a touch of coconut flavor to the soup. Heat the soup over low heat for 2-3 minutes, ensuring it's heated through.
7. Taste and adjust the seasonings as needed, adding more salt and pepper if desired.
8. Ladle the Butternut Squash Soup into serving bowls.
9. For a decorative touch, drizzle a swirl of additional coconut milk on top of each serving and garnish with fresh chives or parsley, if desired.
10. Serve hot, and enjoy your flavorful and nutritious Butternut Squash Soup!

NUTRITIONAL FACTS

Calories: 120 Fat: 4g Protein: 2g Carbs: 24g Sugar: 5g Fiber: 4g Vitamin A: 300% DV

Vitamin C: 50% DV Calcium: 8% DV Iron: 10% DV

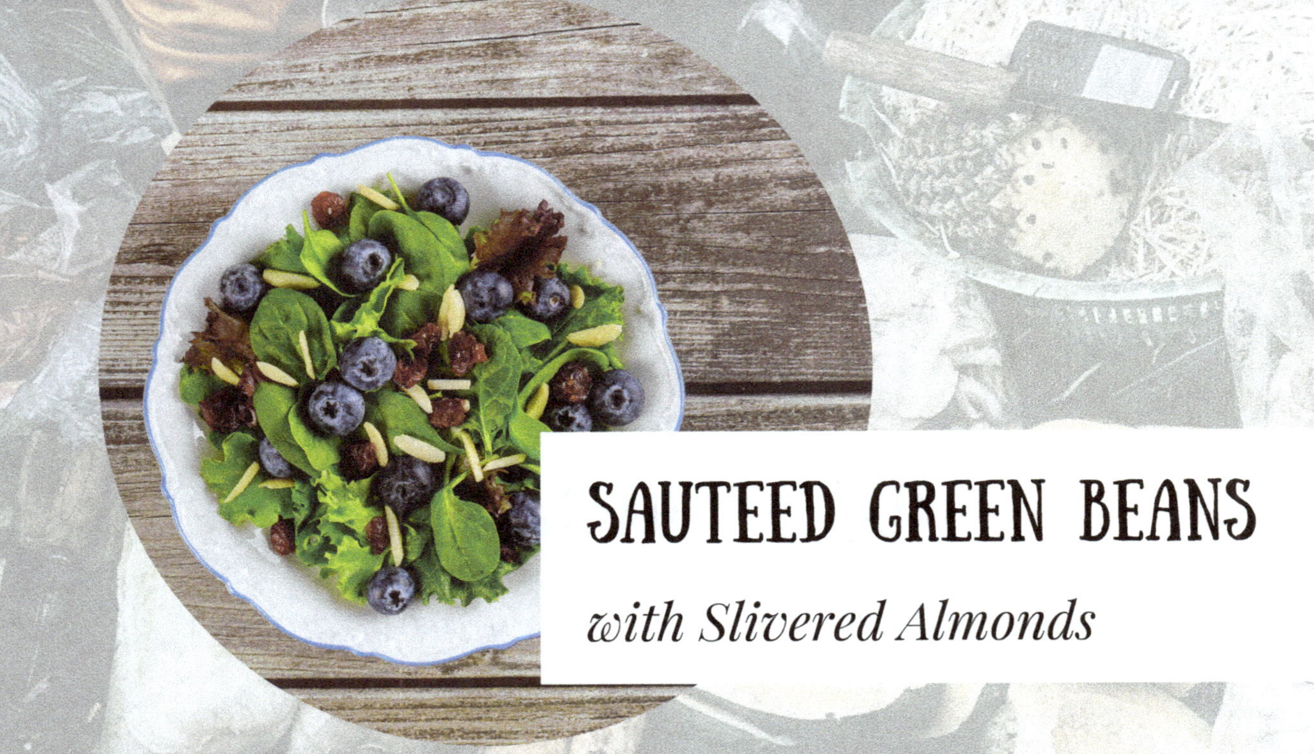

SAUTEED GREEN BEANS

with Slivered Almonds

Prep. Time: 10 minutes | **Cooking Time:** 10 minutes | **Servings:** 4

INGREDIENTS

·1 pound fresh green beans, ends trimmed

·2 tablespoons olive oil

·1/4 cup slivered almonds

·2 cloves garlic, minced

·Salt and pepper to taste

·Zest of 1 lemon (optional)

·Lemon wedges for garnish (optional)

DIRECTIONS

1. Bring a large pot of water to a boil. Add a pinch of salt and the trimmed green beans to the boiling water. Blanch the green beans for about 2-3 minutes until they become bright green and slightly tender but still crisp.

2. Immediately transfer the blanched green beans to a bowl of iced water to stop the cooking process. Drain and set aside.

3. In a large skillet, heat the olive oil over medium-high heat.

4. Add the slivered almonds to the skillet and toast them for 2-3 minutes, stirring frequently, until they turn golden brown. Be careful not to burn them.

5. Add the minced garlic to the skillet and sauté for about 30 seconds until it becomes fragrant.

6. Add the blanched green beans to the skillet. Season with salt and pepper to taste.

7. Saute the green beans for 3-4 minutes, stirring occasionally, until they are heated and have a slight char.

8. If desired, sprinkle the zest of one lemon over the green beans for a burst of citrus flavor.

9. Transfer the Sauteed Green Beans with Slivered Almonds to a serving platter.

10. Garnish with lemon wedges, if desired.

11. Serve hot as a flavorful and nutritious side dish.

NUTRITIONAL FACTS

Calories: 120 Fat: 10g Protein: 3g Carbs: 7g Sugar: 2g Fiber: 3g Vitamin A: 15% DV

Vitamin C: 25% DV Calcium: 6% DV Iron: 10% DV

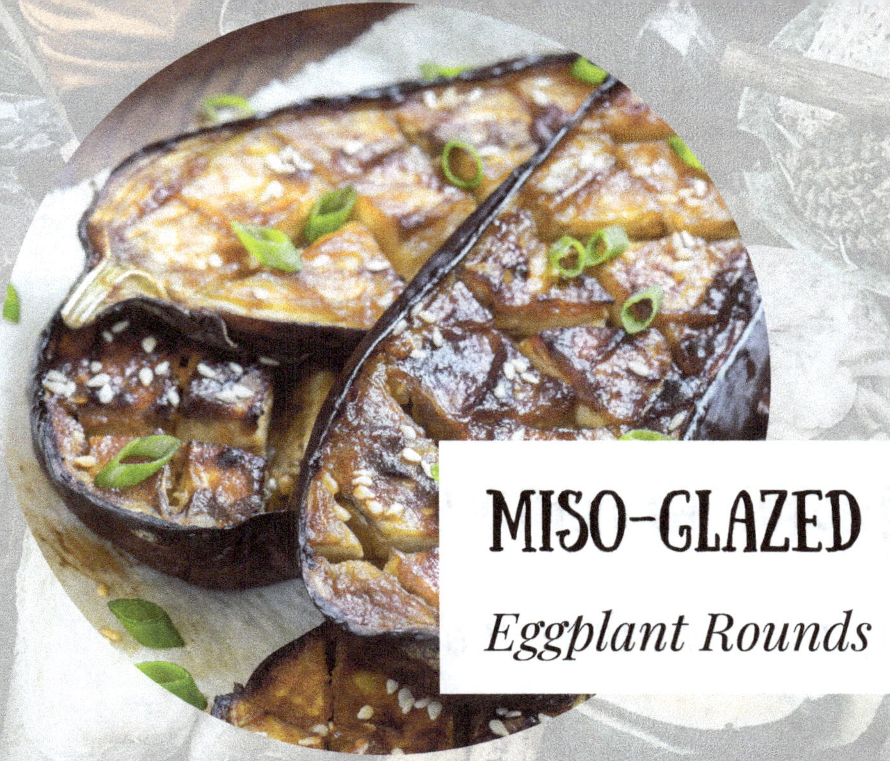

MISO-GLAZED

Eggplant Rounds

Prep. Time: 15 minutes | **Cooking Time:** 10 minutes | **Servings:** 4

INGREDIENTS

- 2 large Japanese or Chinese eggplants
- 2 tablespoons white miso paste
- 1 tablespoon mirin (sweet rice wine)
- 1 tablespoon soy sauce (low-sodium)
- 1 tablespoon rice vinegar
- 1 tablespoon honey or maple syrup
- 1 tablespoon sesame oil
- 2 cloves garlic, minced
- 1 teaspoon grated fresh ginger
- 2 tablespoons chopped fresh cilantro or green onions for garnish (optional)
- Sesame seeds for garnish (optional)

DIRECTIONS

1. Preheat your oven to 400°F (200°C). Line a baking sheet with parchment paper.
2. Slice the eggplants into rounds about 1/2-inch (1.25 cm) thick. Place them in a single layer on the prepared baking sheet.
3. In a small bowl, whisk together the white miso paste, mirin, low-sodium soy sauce, rice vinegar, honey or maple syrup, sesame oil, minced garlic, and grated fresh ginger. This will create the miso glaze.
4. Brush the miso glaze generously over each eggplant round, ensuring they are well coated.
5. Place the baking sheet in the preheated oven and bake for about 15-20 minutes, or until the eggplants are tender and the miso glaze has caramelized and become golden brown.
6. While the eggplants are baking, you can prepare a garnish by chopping fresh cilantro or green onions and toasting sesame seeds if desired.
7. Remove the Miso-Glazed Eggplant Rounds from the oven and transfer them to a serving platter.
8. Garnish with chopped cilantro or green onions and a sprinkle of sesame seeds if you like.
9. Serve hot as a delicious and healthy side dish or appetizer.

NUTRITIONAL FACTS

Calories: 120 Fat: 5g Protein: 2g Carbs: 20g Sugar: 10g Fiber: 5g Vitamin A: 4% DV

Vitamin C: 10% DV Calcium: 2% DV Iron: 4% DV

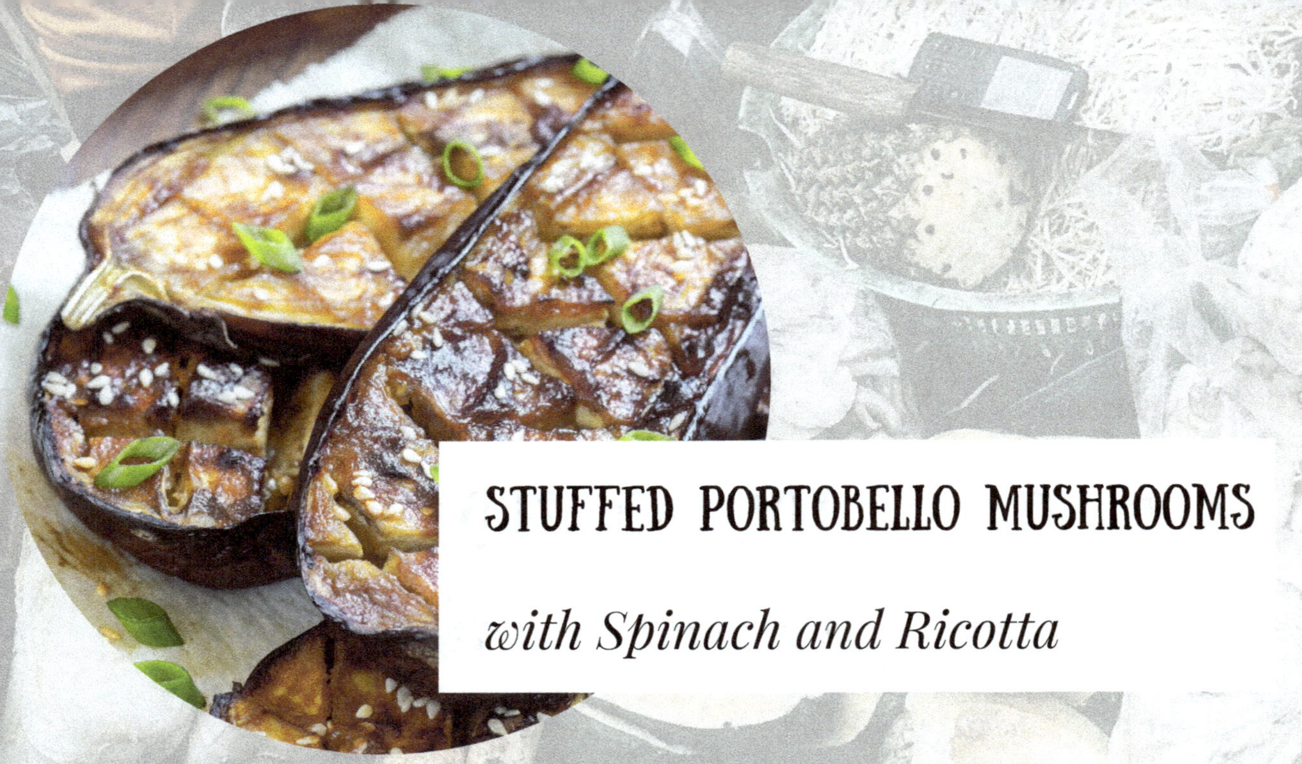

STUFFED PORTOBELLO MUSHROOMS

with Spinach and Ricotta

Prep. Time: 15 minutes | **Cooking Time:** 20 minutes | **Servings:** 4

INGREDIENTS

·4 large Portobello mushrooms, stems removed and cleaned
·2 cups fresh spinach, chopped
·1 cup part-skim ricotta cheese
·1/4 cup grated Parmesan cheese
·2 cloves garlic, minced
·1/2 teaspoon dried oregano
·1/2 teaspoon dried basil
·Salt and pepper to taste
·1 tablespoon olive oil
·Fresh basil leaves for garnish (optional)

DIRECTIONS

1. Preheat your oven to 375°F (190°C). Line a baking sheet with parchment paper.
2. In a large mixing bowl, combine the chopped spinach, ricotta cheese, grated Parmesan cheese, minced garlic, dried oregano, dried basil, salt, and pepper. Mix until all the ingredients are well combined.
3. Place the cleaned Portobello mushrooms on the prepared baking sheet and gill side up.
4. Divide the spinach and ricotta mixture evenly among the Portobello mushrooms, filling the hollows of each mushroom cap.
5. Drizzle the olive oil over the stuffed mushrooms.
6. Place the baking sheet in the oven and bake for about 20 minutes, or until the mushrooms are tender and the stuffing is golden and slightly crispy on top.
7. If desired, garnish the Stuffed Portobello Mushrooms with fresh basil leaves for a pop of color and flavor.
8. Remove the stuffed mushrooms from the oven and transfer them to serving plates.
9. Serve hot as a satisfying and nutrient-rich main course or side dish.

NUTRITIONAL FACTS

Calories: 170 Fat: 9g Protein: 11g Carbs: 10g Sugar: 3g Fiber: 3g Vitamin A: 60% DV
Vitamin C: 20% DV Calcium: 20% DV Iron: 10% DV

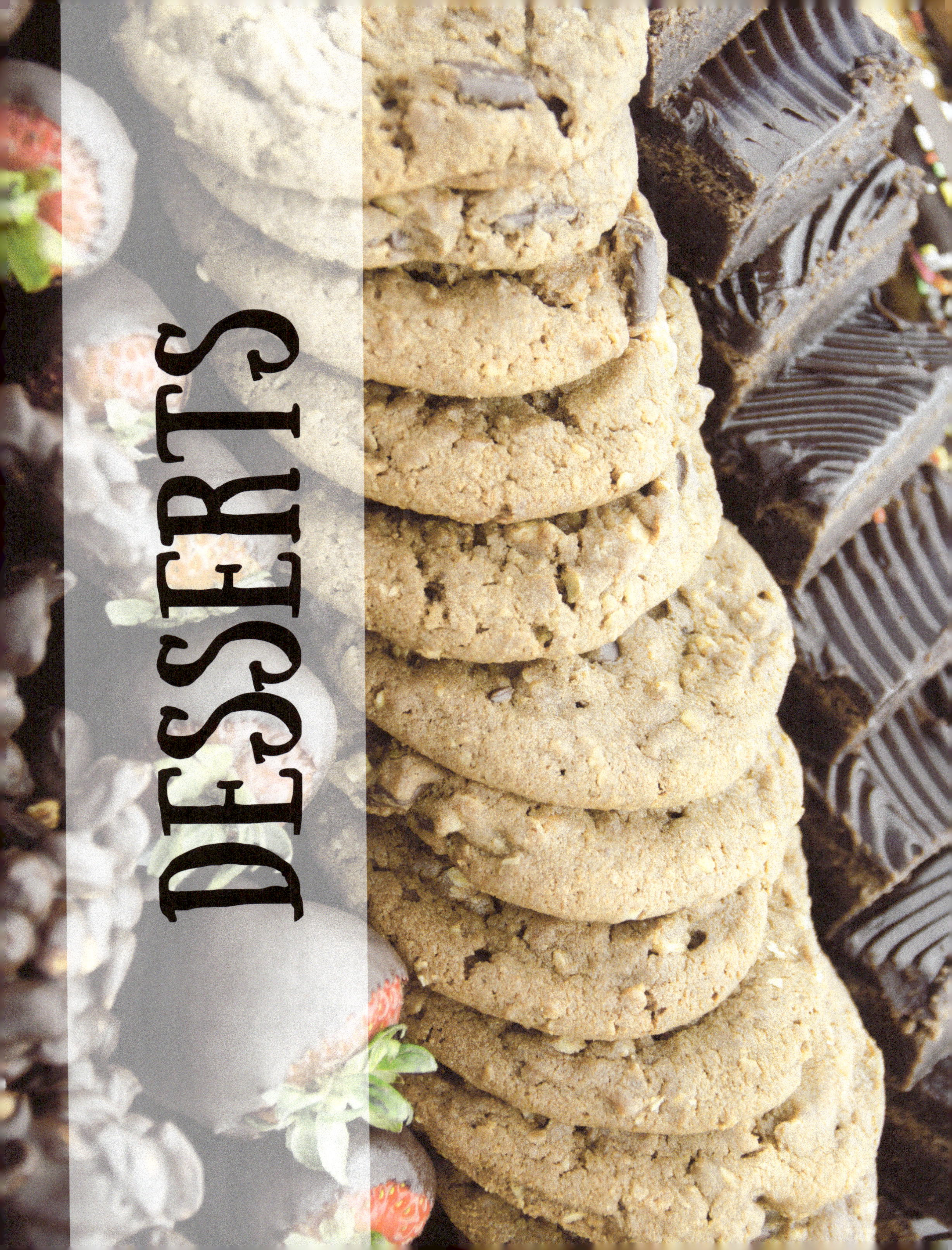

DESSERTS

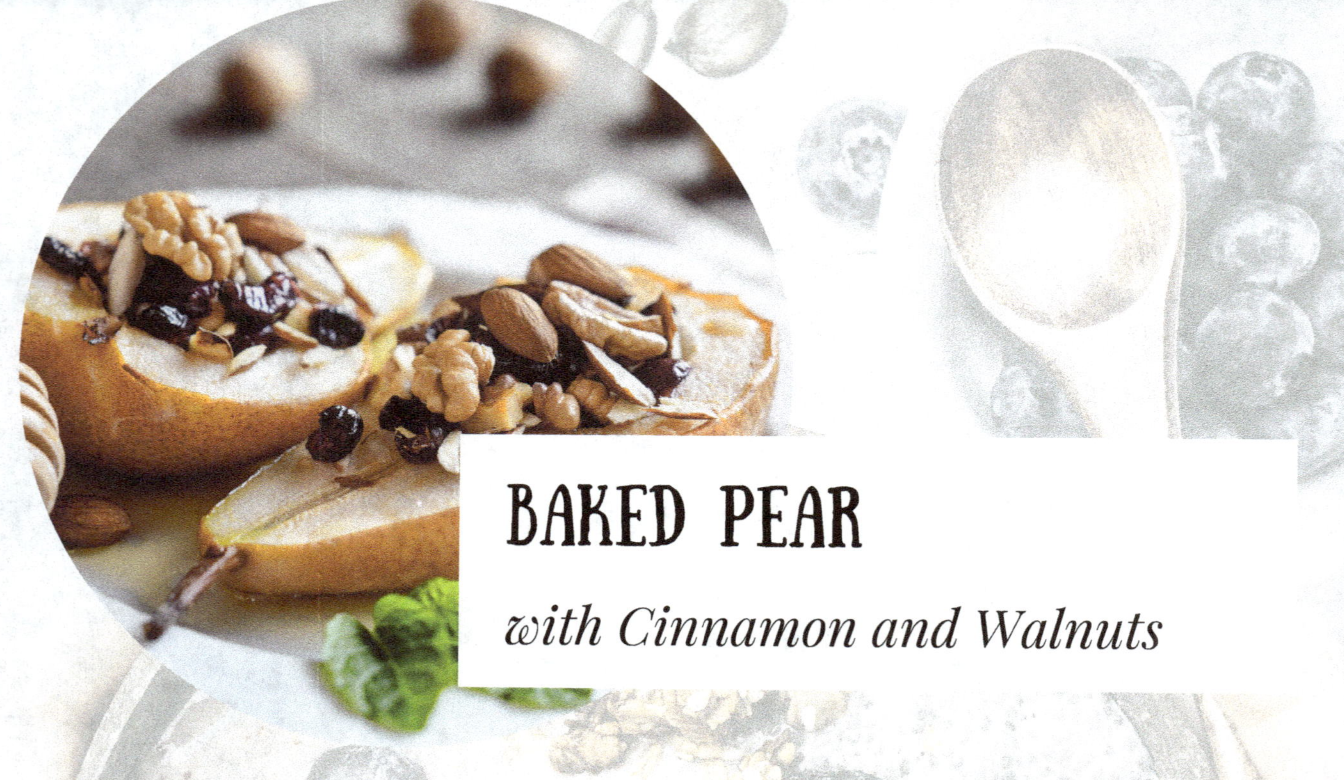

BAKED PEAR

with Cinnamon and Walnuts

Prep. Time: 10 minutes | **Cooking Time:** 25 minutes | **Servings:** 4

INGREDIENTS

- 4 ripe but firm pears
- 2 tablespoons lemon juice
- 2 tablespoons honey
- 1 teaspoon ground cinnamon
- 1/4 cup chopped walnuts

DIRECTIONS

1. Preheat your oven to 375°F (190°C).
2. Wash and peel the pears, leaving the stems intact. Slice a thin layer off the bottom of each pear to create a flat surface so they can stand upright.
3. Cut off the tops of the pears, about 1 inch from the stem end. Set the tops aside.
4. Use a melon baller or a small spoon to scoop out the seeds and core from each pear, creating a hollow cavity.
5. Place the hollowed-out pears in a baking dish.
6. Drizzle the lemon juice over the pears to prevent them from browning.
7. In a small bowl, mix together the honey and ground cinnamon.
8. Spoon the honey-cinnamon mixture into the cavities of the pears, distributing it evenly among them.
9. Sprinkle the chopped walnuts over the tops of the pears.
10. Place the reserved pear tops back on each pear.
11. Add about 1/4 inch of water to the bottom of the baking dish to prevent the pears from sticking.
12. Cover the baking dish with aluminum foil.
13. Bake in the oven for 20-25 minutes or until the pears are tender when pierced with a fork.
14. Remove the foil and bake for 5 minutes to allow the tops to brown slightly.
15. Carefully transfer the baked pears to serving plates.
16. Serve warm, optionally garnished with a drizzle of honey or a sprinkle of cinnamon.

NUTRITIONAL FACTS

Calories: 170 Fat: 5g Protein: 1g Carbs: 39g Sugar: 27g Fiber: 6g Sodium: 1mg Vitamin C: 9% DV Vitamin K: 2% DV Potassium: 219mg Calcium: 2% DV Iron: 2% DV

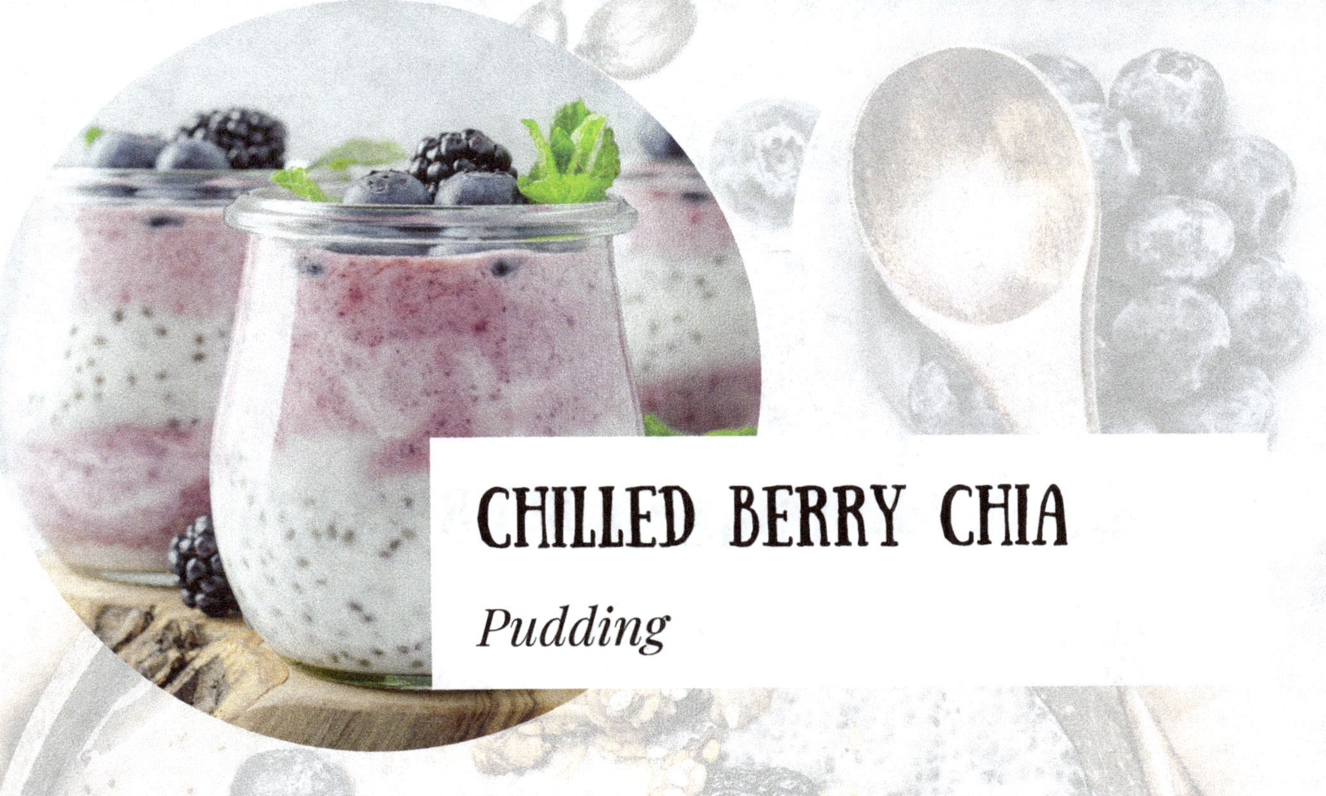

CHILLED BERRY CHIA
Pudding

| **Prep. Time:** 10 minutes | **Chilling Time:** 125 minutes | **Servings:** 4 |

INGREDIENTS

- 1 cup unsweetened almond milk (or any milk of your choice)
- 1/4 cup chia seeds
- 2 tablespoons maple syrup or honey (adjust to taste)
- 1 teaspoon pure vanilla extract
- 1 cup mixed berries (strawberries, blueberries, raspberries)
- Fresh mint leaves for garnish (optional)

DIRECTIONS

1. In a mixing bowl, combine the unsweetened almond milk, chia seeds, maple syrup or honey, and pure vanilla extract.
2. Whisk the mixture well to ensure the chia seeds are evenly distributed. Taste and adjust the sweetness if needed by adding more maple syrup or honey.
3. Cover the bowl and refrigerate for at least 2 hours or overnight. During this time, the chia seeds will absorb the liquid and create a pudding-like consistency.
4. After chilling, give the mixture a good stir to break up any clumps that may have formed.
5. Wash and prepare the mixed berries by slicing the strawberries and leaving smaller berries whole.
6. To serve, divide the chilled chia pudding into four serving cups or glasses.
7. Top each serving with a generous amount of mixed berries.
8. Optionally, garnish with fresh mint leaves for flavor and color.
9. Serve immediately or refrigerate until ready to enjoy.

NUTRITIONAL FACTS

Calories: 120 Fat: 6g Protein: 3g Carbs: 14g Sugar: 6g Fiber: 7g Sodium: 60mg Vitamin C: 20% DV Calcium: 15% DV Iron: 1% DV Potassium: 160mg

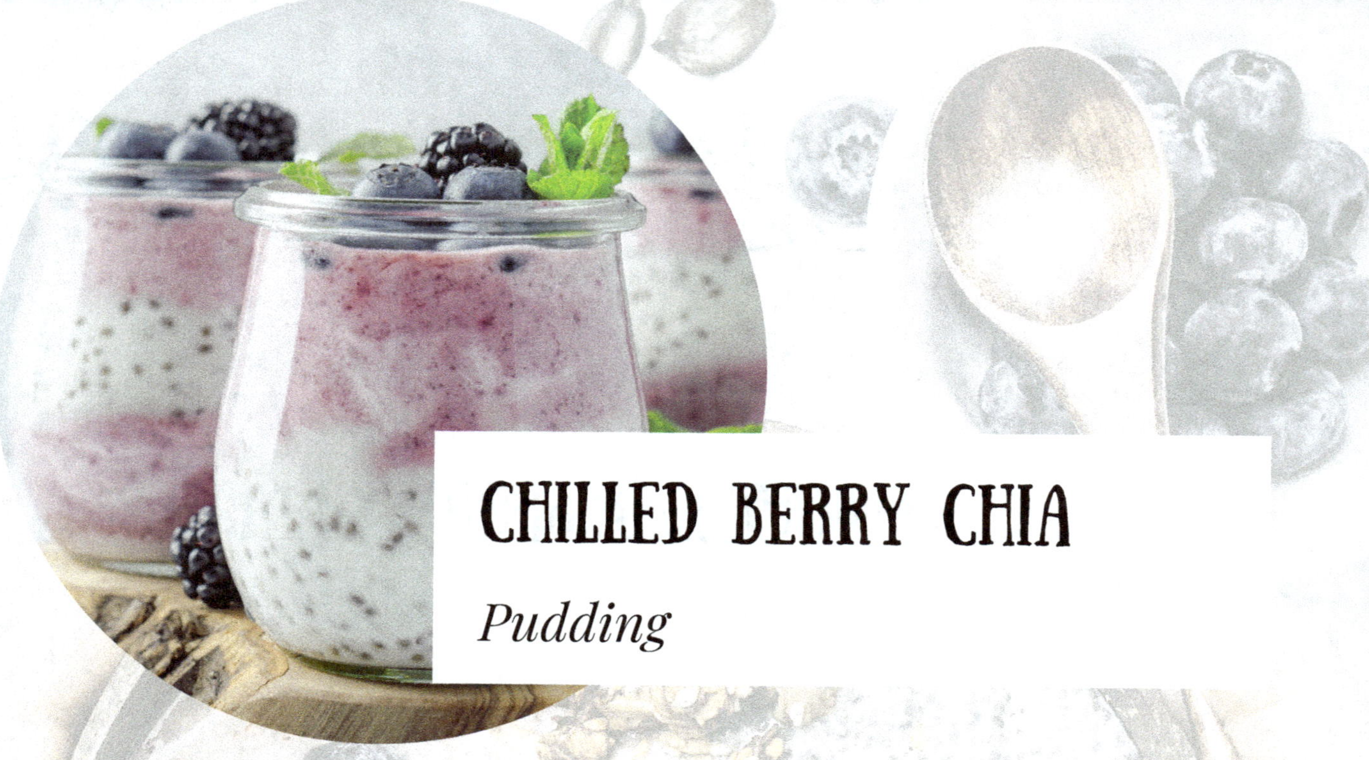

CHILLED BERRY CHIA

Pudding

Prep. Time: 10 minutes | **Chilling Time:** 125 minutes | **Servings:** 4

INGREDIENTS

·1 cup unsweetened almond milk (or any milk of your choice)

·1/4 cup chia seeds

·2 tablespoons maple syrup or honey (adjust to taste)

·1 teaspoon pure vanilla extract

·1 cup mixed berries (strawberries, blueberries, raspberries)

·Fresh mint leaves for garnish (optional)

DIRECTIONS

1. In a mixing bowl, combine the unsweetened almond milk, chia seeds, maple syrup or honey, and pure vanilla extract.
2. Whisk the mixture well to ensure the chia seeds are evenly distributed. Taste and adjust the sweetness if needed by adding more maple syrup or honey.
3. Cover the bowl and refrigerate for at least 2 hours or overnight. During this time, the chia seeds will absorb the liquid and create a pudding-like consistency.
4. After chilling, give the mixture a good stir to break up any clumps that may have formed.
5. Wash and prepare the mixed berries by slicing the strawberries and leaving smaller berries whole.
6. To serve, divide the chilled chia pudding into four serving cups or glasses.
7. Top each serving with a generous amount of mixed berries.
8. Optionally, garnish with fresh mint leaves for flavor and color.
9. Serve immediately or refrigerate until ready to enjoy.

NUTRITIONAL FACTS

Calories: 120 Fat: 6g Protein: 3g Carbs: 14g Sugar: 6g Fiber: 7g Sodium: 60mg Vitamin C: 20% DV Calcium: 15% DV Iron: 1% DV Potassium: 160mg

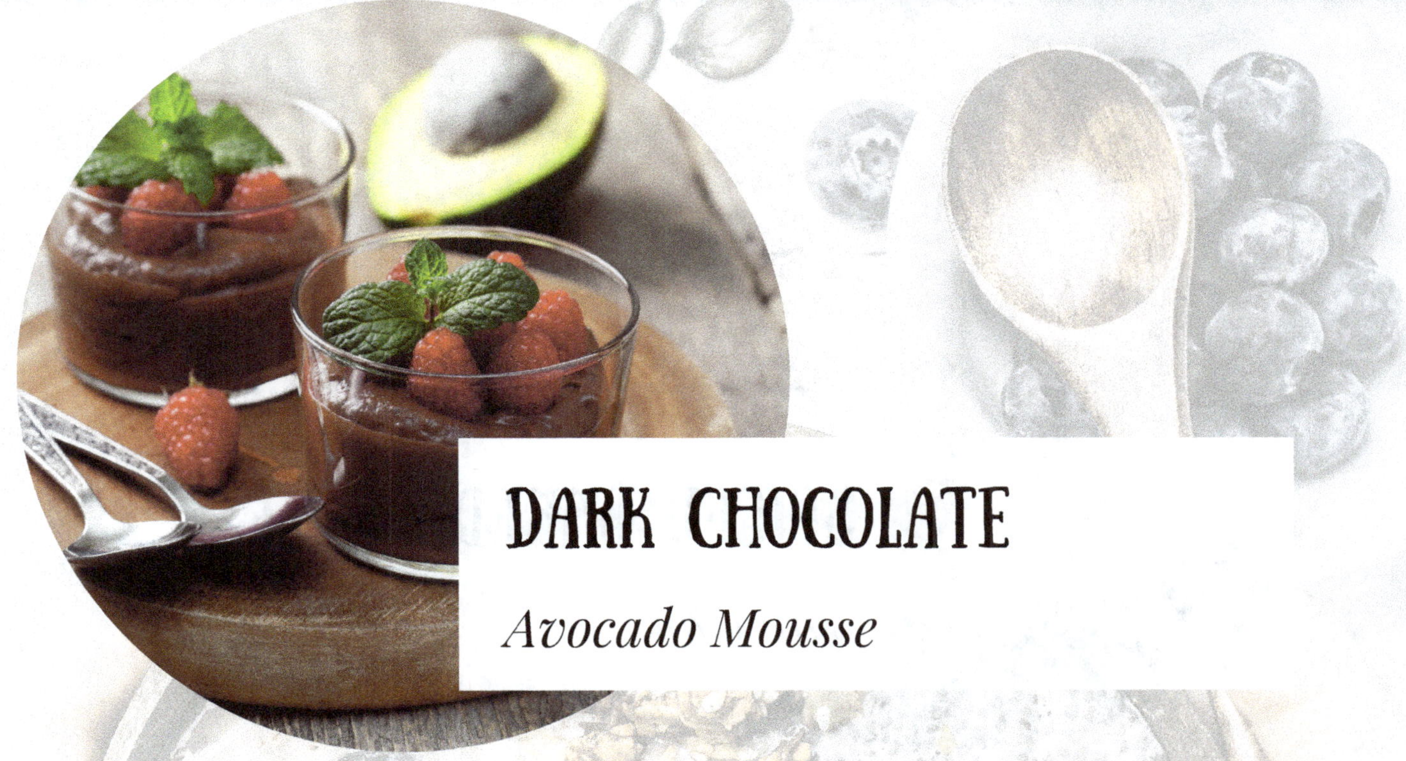

DARK CHOCOLATE

Avocado Mousse

Prep. Time: 10 minutes | **Cooking Time:** / | **Servings:** 4

INGREDIENTS

·2 ripe avocados
·1/4 cup unsweetened cocoa powder
·1/4 cup dark chocolate chips (70% cocoa or higher)
·3 tablespoons maple syrup or honey (adjust to taste)
·1 teaspoon pure vanilla extract
·A pinch of salt
·Fresh berries or mint leaves for garnish (optional)

DIRECTIONS

1. Cut the ripe avocados in half, remove the pits, and scoop the flesh into a food processor.
2. Add unsweetened cocoa powder, dark chocolate chips, maple syrup or honey, pure vanilla extract, and a pinch of salt to the food processor.
3. Blend all the ingredients until smooth and creamy. You may need to stop and scrape down the sides of the food processor a few times to ensure everything is well combined.
4. Taste the mixture and adjust the sweetness by adding more maple syrup or honey if desired.
5. Once the mousse is smooth and sweetened to your liking, spoon it into serving dishes or glasses.
6. Cover and refrigerate for at least 30 minutes to allow it to chill and firm up a bit.
7. Before serving, garnish with fresh berries or mint leaves if desired.
8. Serve and enjoy this delicious and healthy chocolate mousse!

NUTRITIONAL FACTS

Calories: 220 Fat: 16g Protein: 3g Carbs: 21g Sugar: 11g Fiber: 7g Sodium: 10mg Vitamin C: 10% DV Calcium: 2% DV Iron: 10% DV Potassium: 480mg

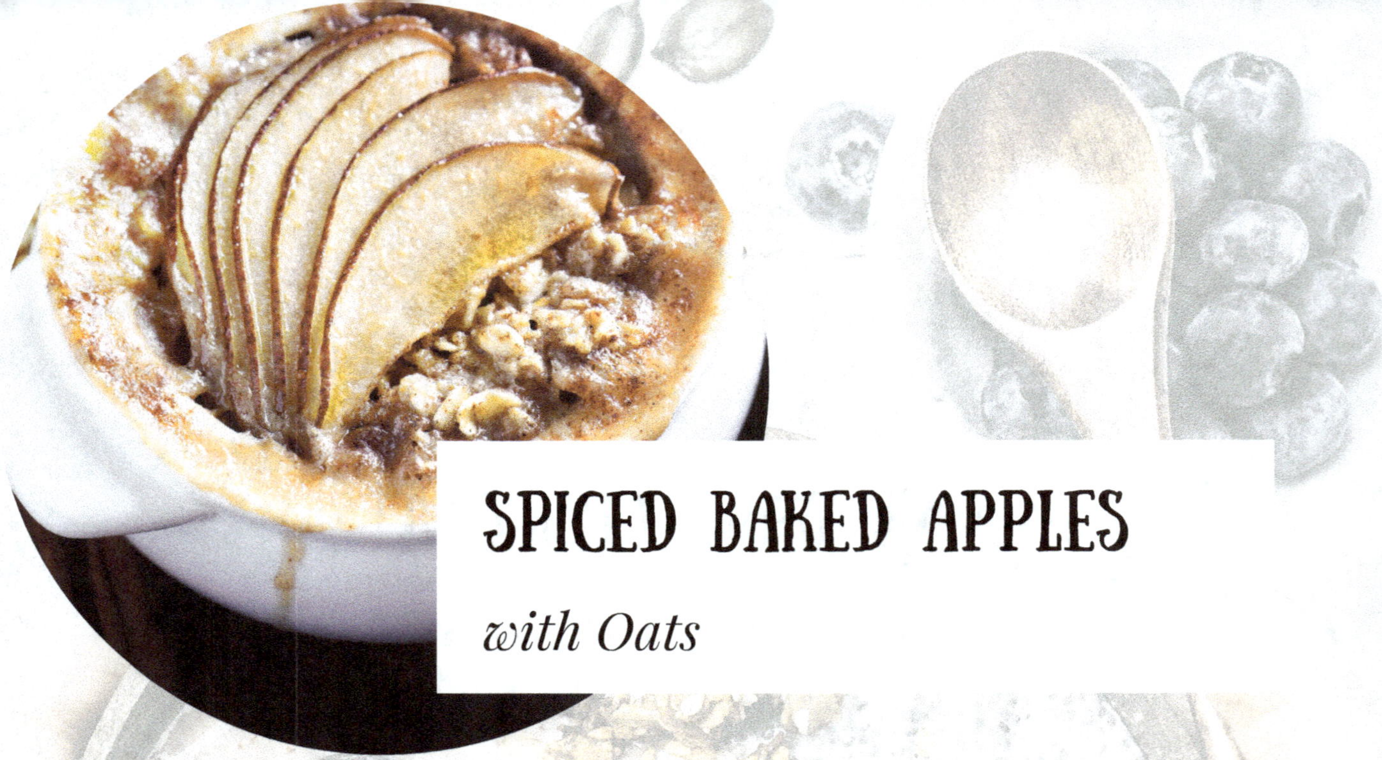

SPICED BAKED APPLES

with Oats

Prep. Time: 10 minutes | **Cooking Time:** / | **Servings:** 4

INGREDIENTS

- 2 ripe avocados
- 1/4 cup unsweetened cocoa powder
- 1/4 cup dark chocolate chips (70% cocoa or higher)
- 3 tablespoons maple syrup or honey (adjust to taste)
- 1 teaspoon pure vanilla extract
- A pinch of salt
- Fresh berries or mint leaves for garnish (optional)

DIRECTIONS

1. Cut the ripe avocados in half, remove the pits, and scoop the flesh into a food processor.
2. Add unsweetened cocoa powder, dark chocolate chips, maple syrup or honey, pure vanilla extract, and a pinch of salt to the food processor.
3. Blend all the ingredients until smooth and creamy. You may need to stop and scrape down the sides of the food processor a few times to ensure everything is well combined.
4. Taste the mixture and adjust the sweetness by adding more maple syrup or honey if desired.
5. Once the mousse is smooth and sweetened to your liking, spoon it into serving dishes or glasses.
6. Cover and refrigerate for at least 30 minutes to allow it to chill and firm up a bit.
7. Before serving, garnish with fresh berries or mint leaves if desired.
8. Serve and enjoy this delicious and healthy chocolate mousse!

NUTRITIONAL FACTS

Calories: 220 Fat: 16g Protein: 3g Carbs: 21g Sugar: 11g Fiber: 7g Sodium: 10mg Vitamin C: 10% DV Calcium: 2% DV Iron: 10% DV Potassium: 480mg

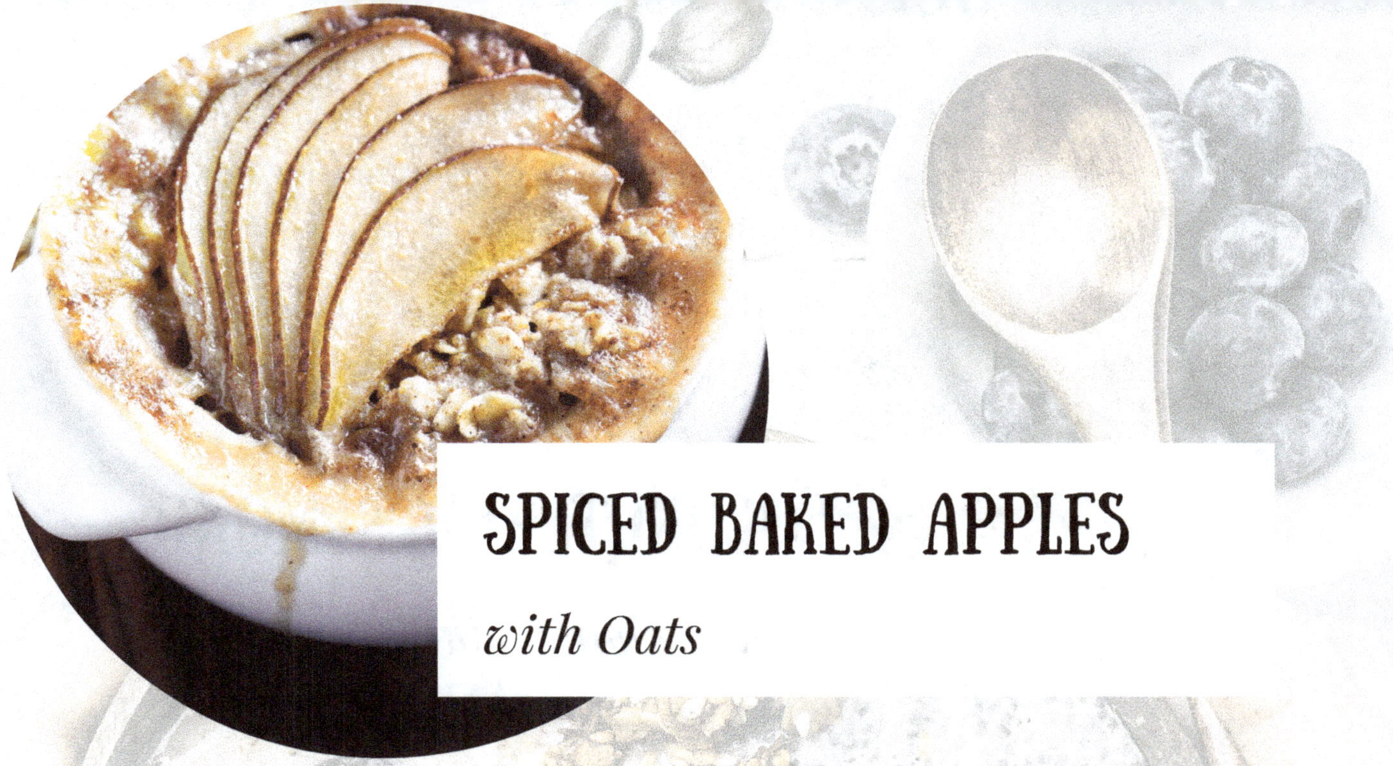

SPICED BAKED APPLES

with Oats

Prep. Time: 15 minutes | **Cooking Time:** 25 minutes | **Servings:** 4

INGREDIENTS

·4 medium-sized apples (such as Granny Smith or Honeycrisp)

·1/2 cup rolled oats

·1/4 cup chopped nuts (e.g., walnuts or pecans)

·2 tablespoons maple syrup or honey

·1 tablespoon melted coconut oil or butter

·1 teaspoon ground cinnamon

·1/4 teaspoon ground nutmeg

·1/4 teaspoon ground cloves

·A pinch of salt

·Greek yogurt or vanilla ice cream for serving (optional)

DIRECTIONS

1. Preheat your oven to 350°F (175°C).

2. Wash the apples and carefully core them using a knife or an apple corer, leaving the bottom intact to create a well for the filling. Place the cored apples in a baking dish.

3. In a mixing bowl, combine rolled oats, chopped nuts, maple syrup or honey, melted coconut oil or butter, ground cinnamon, ground nutmeg, ground cloves, and a pinch of salt. Mix everything together until the mixture is well combined.

4. Spoon the oat and nut mixture into the cavities of the cored apples, pressing down gently to pack the filling.

5. Cover the baking dish with foil and bake in the oven for 20 minutes.

6. After 20 minutes, remove the foil and bake for 5-10 minutes, or until the apples are tender and the oat topping is golden brown.

7. Remove the baked apples from the oven and let them cool slightly.

8. Serve the spiced baked apples with a dollop of Greek yogurt or a scoop of vanilla ice cream if desired.

9. Enjoy your delicious and wholesome dessert!

NUTRITIONAL FACTS

Calories: 235 Fat: 10g Protein: 4g Carbs: 38g Sugar: 22g Fiber: 6g Sodium: 55mg Vitamin C: 14% DV Calcium: 3% DV Iron: 7% DV Potassium: 276mg

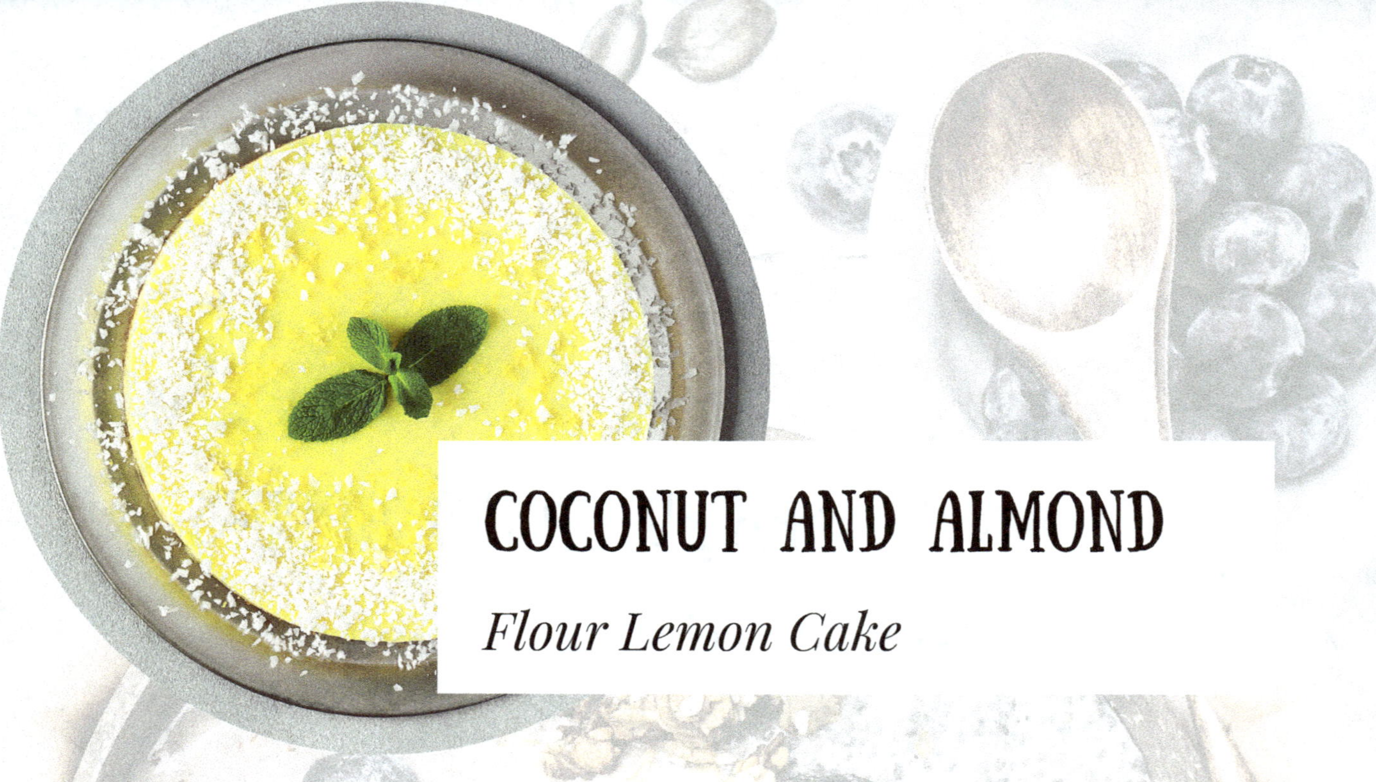

COCONUT AND ALMOND
Flour Lemon Cake

Prep. Time: 15 minutes | **Cooking Time:** 30 minutes | **Servings:** 8

INGREDIENTS

- 1 cup almond flour
- 1/4 cup coconut flour
- 1/2 cup unsweetened shredded coconut
- 1/2 cup granulated erythritol or your preferred sugar substitute
- 1/2 teaspoon baking powder
- 1/4 teaspoon salt
- 4 large eggs
- 1/4 cup unsweetened almond milk
- 1/4 cup melted coconut oil
- Zest and juice of 1 lemon
- 1 teaspoon pure vanilla extract

For the Lemon Glaze:
- 1/4 cup powdered erythritol or powdered sugar substitute
- Juice of 1 lemon

DIRECTIONS

1. Preheat your oven to 350°F (175°C). Grease an 8-inch round cake pan and line the bottom with parchment paper for easy removal.
2. In a mixing bowl, whisk together the almond flour, coconut flour, shredded coconut, granulated erythritol, baking powder, and salt.
3. In another bowl, whisk the eggs, almond milk, melted coconut oil, lemon zest, lemon juice, and vanilla extract until well combined.
4. Pour the wet ingredients into the dry ingredients and stir until you have a smooth batter.
5. Pour the batter into the prepared cake pan and spread it evenly.
6. Bake in the preheated oven for about 25-30 minutes or until a toothpick inserted into the center comes out clean, and the top is golden brown.
7. While the cake is baking, prepare the lemon glaze. In a small bowl, mix the powdered erythritol (or powdered sugar substitute) with the lemon juice until you have a smooth glaze.
8. Once the cake is done, remove it from the oven and let it cool in the pan for a few minutes. Then, transfer it to a wire rack to cool completely.
9. Drizzle the lemon glaze over the cooled cake.
10. Slice and serve your delicious coconut and almond flour lemon cake.

NUTRITIONAL FACTS

Calories: 210 Fat: 17g Protein: 5g Carbs: 8g Sugar: 2g Fiber: 3g Sodium: 115mg Vitamin C: 8% DV Calcium: 5% DV Iron: 6% DV Potassium: 91mg

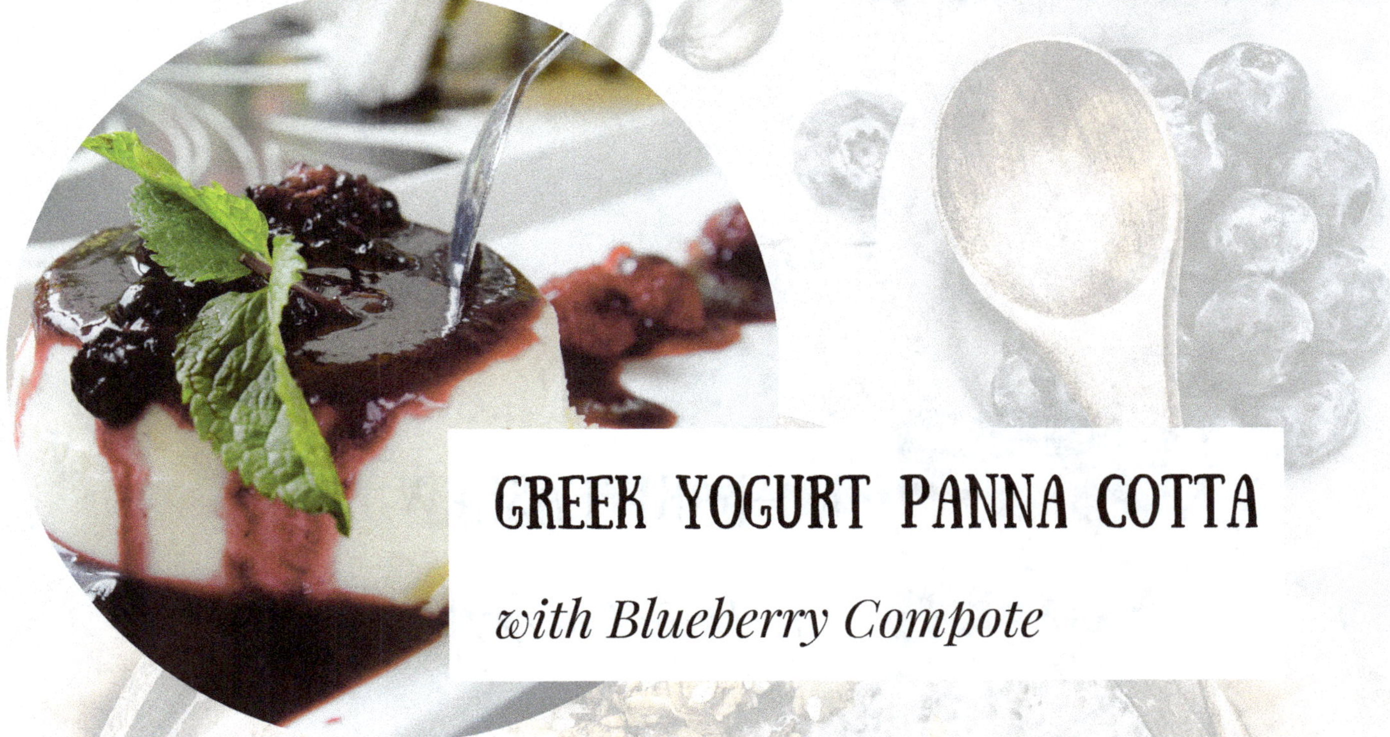

GREEK YOGURT PANNA COTTA

with Blueberry Compote

Prep. Time: 15 minutes | **Cooking Time:** 10 minutes | **Servings:** 8

INGREDIENTS

For the Panna Cotta:
- 2 cups plain Greek yogurt
- 1/2 cup unsweetened almond milk (or your preferred milk)
- 1/4 cup honey or a sugar substitute
- 1 teaspoon pure vanilla extract
- 2 teaspoons unflavored gelatin powder
- 2 tablespoons cold water

For the Blueberry Compote:
- 1 cup fresh or frozen blueberries
- 2 tablespoons water
- 1 tablespoon honey or a sugar substitute
- 1/2 teaspoon lemon zest
- 1 teaspoon lemon juice

DIRECTIONS

1. In a small bowl, combine the unflavored gelatin powder and cold water. Let it sit for a few minutes to bloom.
2. In a saucepan over low heat, warm the almond milk (or your preferred milk) until it's just steaming but not boiling.
3. In a separate mixing bowl, whisk together the Greek yogurt, honey (or sugar substitute), and vanilla extract until well combined.
4. Slowly pour the warm almond milk into the yogurt mixture, whisking continuously until smooth.
5. Microwave the bloomed gelatin for about 10 seconds or until it becomes liquid. Make sure it's not hot.
6. Pour the gelatin mixture into the yogurt mixture and whisk until fully incorporated.
7. Divide the panna cotta mixture among four serving glasses or ramekins.
8. Refrigerate the panna cotta for at least 4 hours or until it's set.
9. While the panna cotta is chilling, prepare the blueberry compote. In a small saucepan, combine the blueberries, water, honey (or sugar substitute), lemon zest, and lemon juice.
10. Cook over medium heat, stirring occasionally, until the blueberries break down and the mixture thickens slightly, about 8-10 minutes.
11. Remove the compote from the heat and let it cool to room temperature.
12. Once the panna cotta is set, spoon the blueberry compote on top of each serving.
13. Chill for an additional 30 minutes to allow the compote to set.
14. Serve your Greek Yogurt Panna Cotta with Blueberry Compote chilled.

NUTRITIONAL FACTS

Calories: 240 Fat: 6g Protein: 14g Carbs: 34g Sugar: 26g Fiber: 2g Sodium: 75mg Vitamin C: 6% DV Calcium: 15% DV Iron: 2% DV

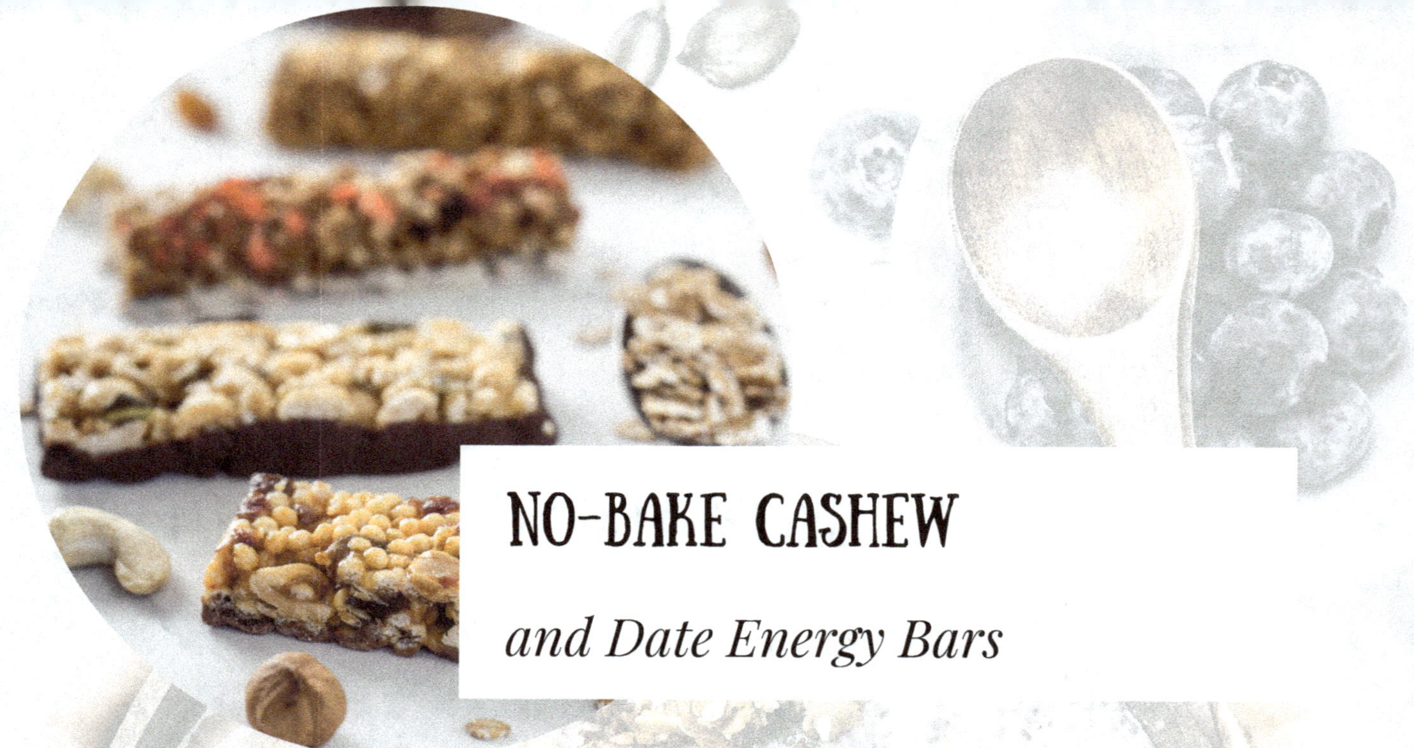

NO-BAKE CASHEW

and Date Energy Bars

Prep. Time: 15 minutes | **Cooking Time:** / | **Servings:** 12

INGREDIENTS

- 1 cup pitted Medjool dates (about 12-14 dates)
- 1 cup raw cashews
- 1/2 cup rolled oats
- 1/4 cup unsweetened shredded coconut
- 2 tablespoons honey or maple syrup
- 1/2 teaspoon pure vanilla extract
- A pinch of salt

DIRECTIONS

1. Place the pitted Medjool dates in a bowl of warm water and let them soak for 5-10 minutes to soften.
2. In a food processor, add the raw cashews, rolled oats, and unsweetened shredded coconut. Pulse until you have a coarse, crumbly texture.
3. Drain the soaked dates and add them to the food processor with honey (or maple syrup), pure vanilla extract, and a pinch of salt.
4. Process the mixture until it starts to come together into a sticky dough. Stop and scrape down the sides of the food processor a few times.
5. Line an 8x8-inch (20x20 cm) baking pan with parchment paper, leaving some overhang on the sides for easy removal.
6. Transfer the dough mixture to the lined pan. Use a spatula or your hands to press it firmly and evenly into the pan.
7. Place the pan in the refrigerator for 30 minutes to firm up.
8. Once the mixture has chilled and set, use the parchment paper overhangs to lift the block out of the pan. Place it on a cutting board.
9. Use a sharp knife to cut the block into 12 equal-sized bars.
10. Store the No-Bake Cashew and Date Energy Bars in an airtight container in the refrigerator for up to two weeks.

NUTRITIONAL FACTS

Calories: 160 Fat: 7g Protein: 3g Carbs: 24g Sugar: 16g Fiber: 2g Sodium: 2mg Iron: 1mg Calcium: 13mg Potassium: 210mg

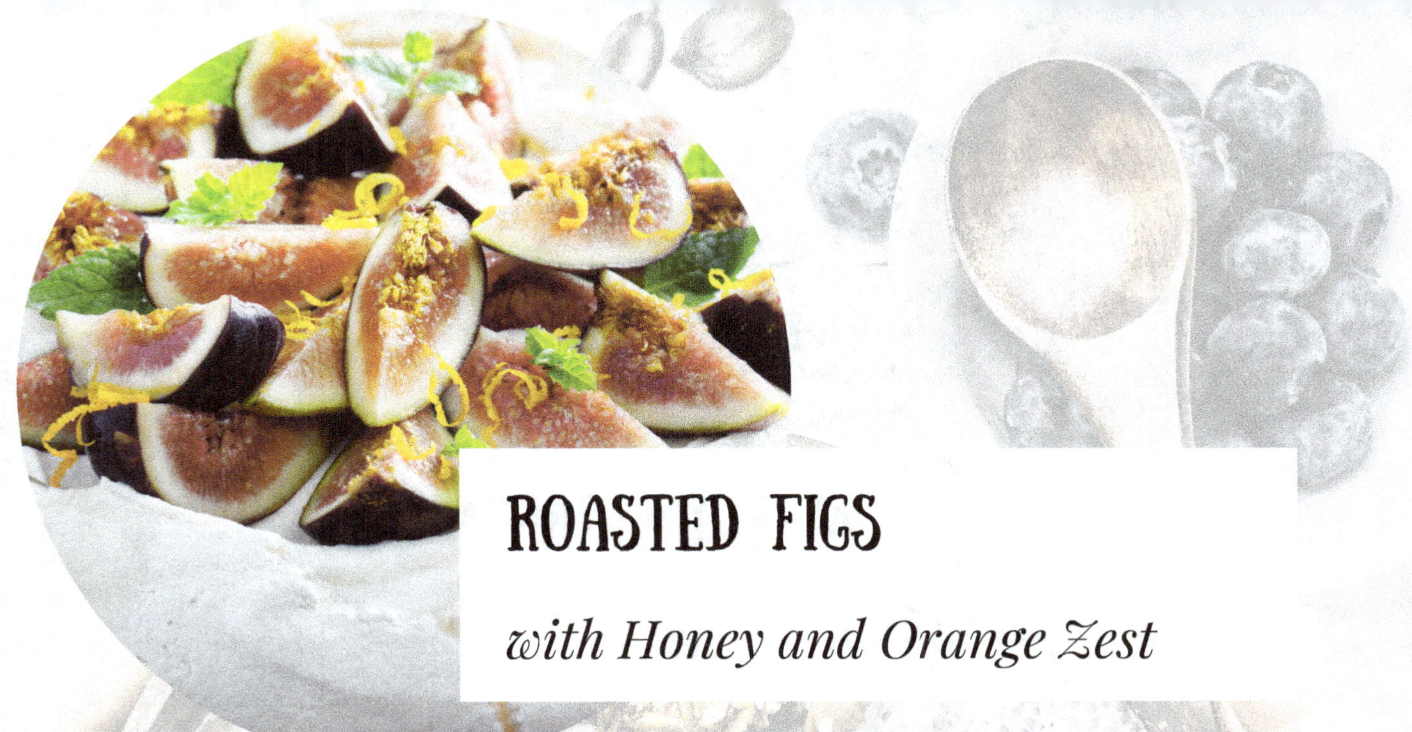

ROASTED FIGS

with Honey and Orange Zest

Prep. Time: 10 minutes | **Cooking Time:** 10 minutes | **Servings:** 4

INGREDIENTS

·12 fresh figs, stemmed and
halved

·2 tablespoons honey

·Zest of 1 orange

·1 tablespoon fresh orange
juice (optional)

·1/4 teaspoon ground
cinnamon

·A pinch of salt

·Cooking spray or olive oil for
greasing

DIRECTIONS

1. Preheat your oven to 400°F (200°C).
2. Slice the fresh figs in half lengthwise and set them aside.
3. In a small bowl, combine the honey, orange zest, fresh orange juice (if using), ground cinnamon, and a pinch of salt. Mix well to create a glaze.
4. Place the halved figs on a baking sheet lined with parchment paper or lightly greased with cooking spray or olive oil.
5. Drizzle the honey and orange zest glaze evenly over the fig halves, ensuring they are well coated.
6. Place the baking sheet in the oven and roast the figs for about 10 minutes or until they become soft and slightly caramelized.
7. Remove the roasted figs from the oven and let them cool slightly.
8. Serve the Roasted Figs with Honey and Orange Zest as a delightful snack or dessert option. You can also pair them with a dollop of Greek yogurt for added creaminess.

NUTRITIONAL FACTS

Calories: 94 Fat: 0.2g Protein: 1g Carbs: 24g Sugar: 21g Fiber: 3g Sodium: 0.6mg Vitamin C: 9mg Calcium: 35mg Iron: 0.4mg Potassium: 238mg

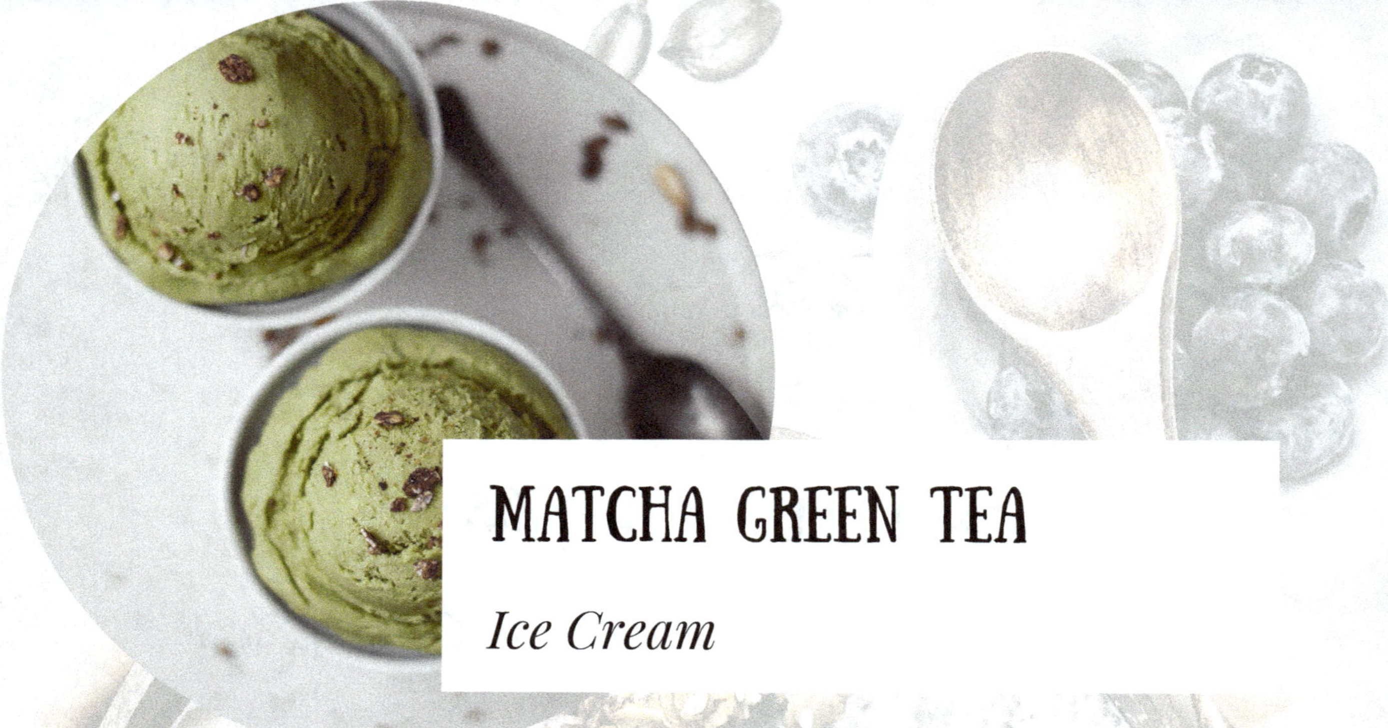

MATCHA GREEN TEA

Ice Cream

Prep. Time: 15 minutes | **Cooking Time:** / | **Servings:** 6

INGREDIENTS

- ·2 cups heavy cream
- ·1 cup whole milk
- ·3/4 cup granulated sugar
- ·3 tablespoons high-quality matcha green tea powder
- ·1 teaspoon vanilla extract
- ·A pinch of salt
- ·4 large egg yolks

DIRECTIONS

1. In a medium mixing bowl, whisk together the matcha green tea powder and granulated sugar until well combined.
2. In a separate saucepan, heat the heavy cream and whole milk over medium heat. Stir occasionally until it begins to steam and is just about to simmer. Do not let it boil.
3. While the cream mixture is heating, in another bowl, whisk the egg yolks until they become slightly pale in color.
4. Once the cream mixture is steaming, gradually add about half to the matcha sugar mixture, whisking continuously to combine.
5. Pour the matcha cream mixture back into the saucepan with the remaining cream mixture. Cook over low to medium-low heat, stirring constantly, until the mixture thickens and coats the back of a spoon. This should take about 5-7 minutes. Do not let it boil.
6. Remove the saucepan from the heat and strain the mixture through a fine-mesh sieve into a clean bowl to remove any potential lumps.
7. Stir in the vanilla extract and a pinch of salt. Let the mixture cool to room temperature, and then cover it and refrigerate it for at least 4 hours or overnight.
8. Once the matcha ice cream base is thoroughly chilled, churn it in your maker according to the manufacturer's instructions.
9. Transfer the churned ice cream to an airtight container and freeze it for 2-4 hours or until it reaches the desired firmness.
10. Serve your homemade Matcha Green Tea Ice Cream in small scoops, and enjoy!

NUTRITIONAL FACTS

Calories: 366 Fat: 27g Protein: 4g Carbs: 29g Sugar: 24g Fiber: 0g Sodium: 49mg Vitamin C: 1mg Calcium: 103mg Iron: 1mg

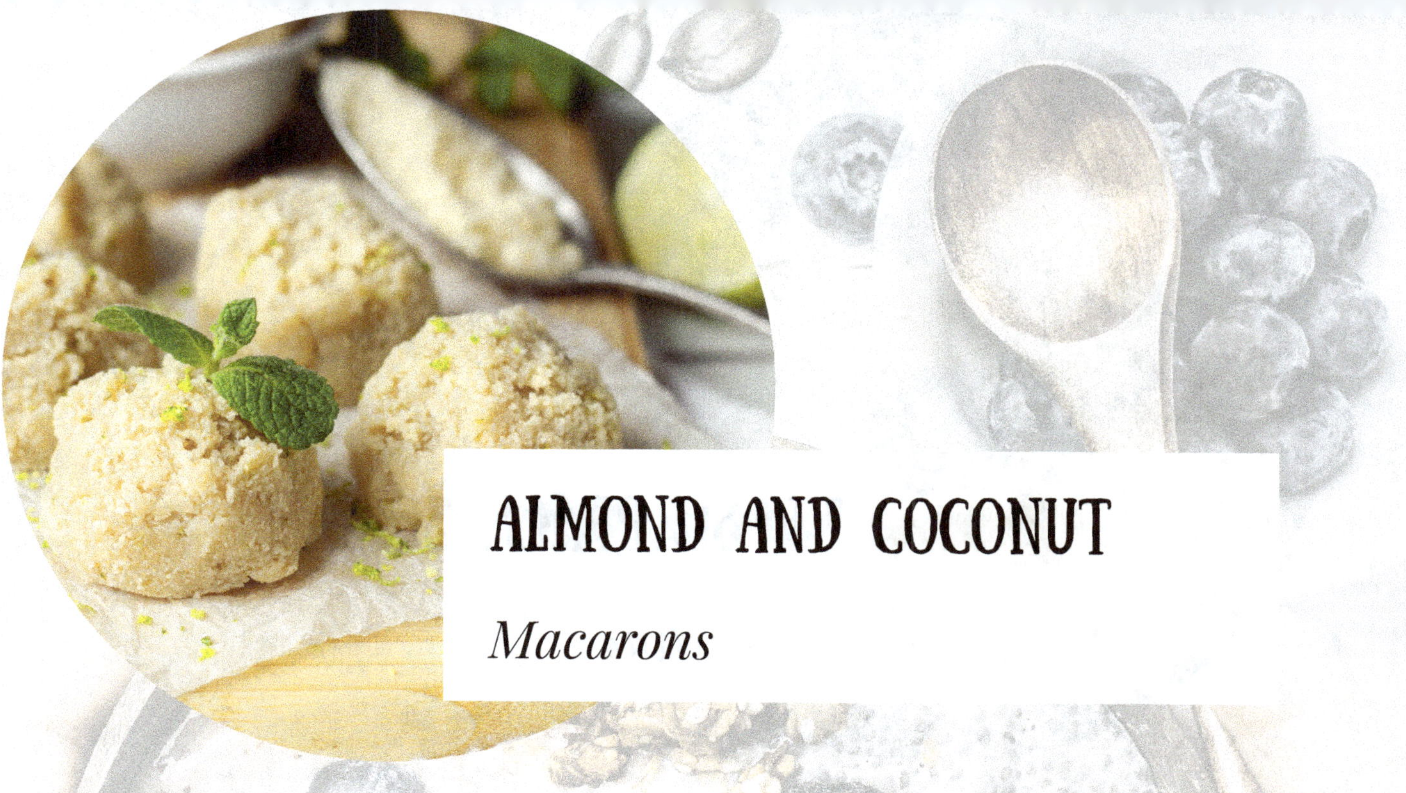

ALMOND AND COCONUT

Macarons

Prep. Time: 15 minutes | **Cooking Time:** 20 minutes | **Servings:** 20 pz

INGREDIENTS

- 2 cups shredded unsweetened coconut
- 1 cup almond flour
- 1/2 cup granulated erythritol or sweetener of your choice
- 2 large egg whites
- 1/4 teaspoon almond extract
- 1/4 teaspoon vanilla extract
- A pinch of salt

DIRECTIONS

1. Preheat your oven to 325°F (160°C). Line a baking sheet with parchment paper.
2. In a large mixing bowl, combine the shredded unsweetened coconut, almond flour, and granulated erythritol. Mix well.
3. In a separate bowl, whisk the egg whites until they become frothy and stiffen.
4. Gently fold the frothy egg whites into the dry mixture until well combined. Be careful not to deflate the egg whites too much; they should provide some lift to the macaroons.
5. Stir in the almond extract, vanilla extract, and a pinch of salt. Mix until the ingredients are evenly distributed.
6. Using a spoon or a cookie scoop, portion out small mounds of the mixture onto the prepared baking sheet. You should be able to make about 20 macaroons.
7. Bake in the oven for 18–20 minutes or until the macaroons are golden brown outside.
8. Remove the macaroons from the oven and let them cool on the baking sheet for a few minutes before transferring them to a wire rack to cool completely.
9. Once the macaroons are excellent, they are ready to enjoy.

NUTRITIONAL FACTS

Calories: 82 Fat: 7g Protein: 2g Carbs: 4g Sugar: 1g Fiber: 2g Sodium: 25mg Calcium: 13mg Iron: 1mg

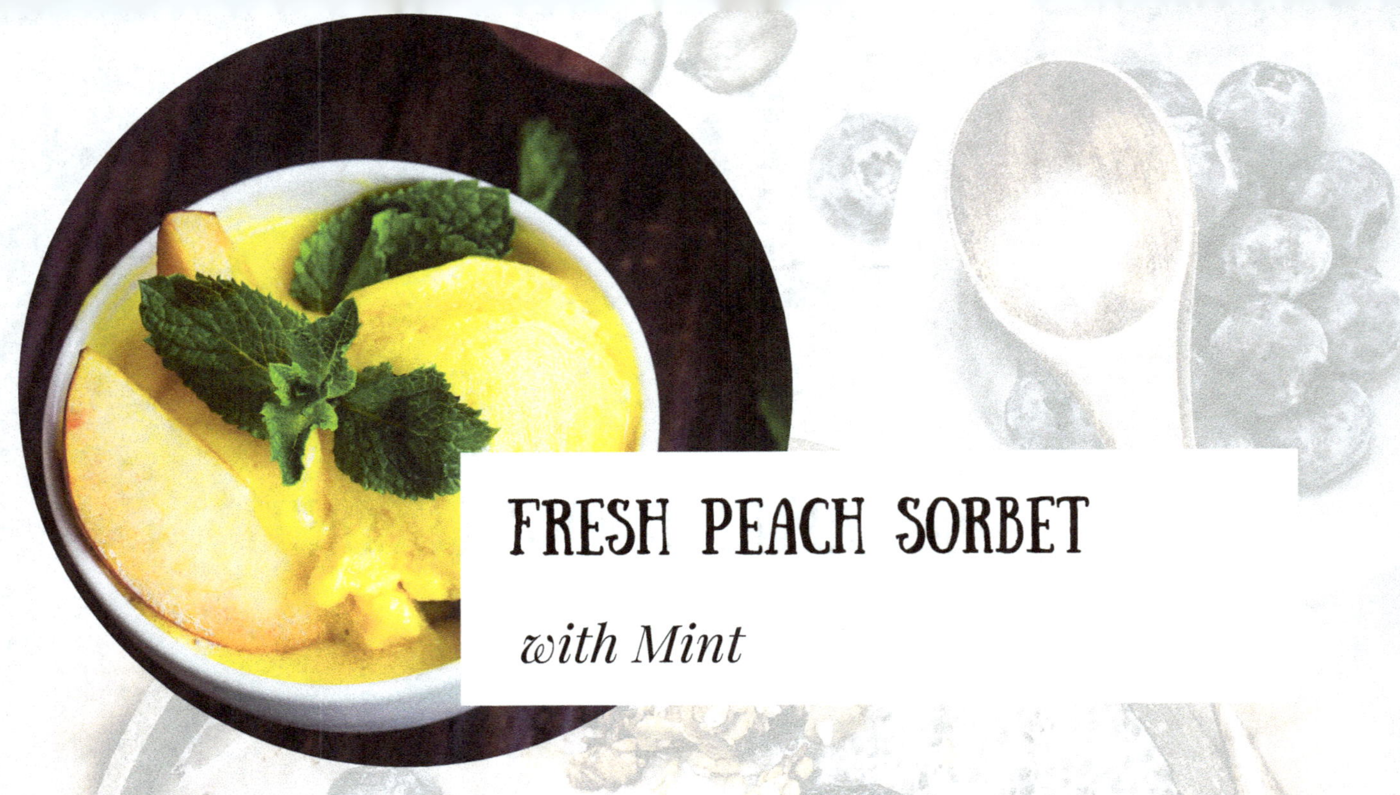

FRESH PEACH SORBET

with Mint

Prep. Time: 10 minutes | **Cooking Time:** / | **Servings:** 4

INGREDIENTS

·4 ripe peaches, peeled, pitted, and sliced

·1/4 cup fresh mint leaves

·1/4 cup granulated erythritol or sweetener of your choice (adjust to taste)

·1 tablespoon fresh lemon juice

·1/2 teaspoon vanilla extract

·A pinch of salt

DIRECTIONS

1. Start by peeling, pitting, and slicing the ripe peaches. If your peaches are not very sweet, you can add a bit more sweetener to taste.

2. In a blender or food processor, combine the sliced peaches, fresh mint leaves, granulated erythritol (or sweetener of your choice), fresh lemon juice, vanilla extract, and a pinch of salt.

3. Blend the mixture until it becomes smooth and well combined. You may need to stop and scrape down the sides of the blender or food processor to ensure everything is evenly mixed.

4. Taste the sorbet mixture and adjust the sweetness or mint flavor to your preference by adding more sweetener or mint leaves if necessary. Blend again to incorporate any additional ingredients.

5. Once the sorbet mixture is smooth and suits your taste, transfer it to an airtight container and place it in the freezer for about 2-3 hours or until it's firm.

6. After the sorbet has hardened, you can use an ice cream scoop or spoon to serve it in bowls or glasses. Garnish with additional mint leaves if desired.

NUTRITIONAL FACTS

Calories: 71 Fat: 0.5g Protein: 1g Carbs: 18g Sugar: 13g Fiber: 2g Sodium: 0mg Vitamin C: 10mg Calcium: 11mg Iron: 0.3mg

CONCLUSION

Dear Reader,

You have reached the end of this journey together, a path I hope has been as enlightening for you as it has been for me to share it. Intermittent fasting is not just a dietary practice, but a step towards greater self-awareness and understanding of your body, especially in this wonderful stage of life.

Remember, every step you have taken in reading this book is a sign of your strength and commitment to deeper well-being. Whether you are at the beginning of your journey with intermittent fasting or have already made significant strides, I want to congratulate you for the courage and determination you have shown.

This path you have embarked on is as personal as it is powerful. It is a testament to your desire to take care of yourself, to listen to your body, and to nourish it in the most conscious and respectful way. Each day that you apply the principles of intermittent fasting, you are making a positive choice for your health and well-being, a choice that will reflect in every aspect of your life.

Don't forget that the journey towards well-being is a continuous one, full of discoveries and moments of growth. There is much to learn from every experience, be it successes or challenges. Be patient with yourself and celebrate every small achievement. Your journey is unique, just like you.

Before closing, I would like to ask you a small favor. If you found this book helpful, I would be immensely grateful if you could leave an honest review. Your feedback will not only help me improve but will also help other women like you to discover and benefit from this extraordinary path.

I wish you all the best, a life full of serenity, and a continuous journey towards well-being. Thank you for sharing this journey with me.

With affection and gratitude,

Hanna Holden

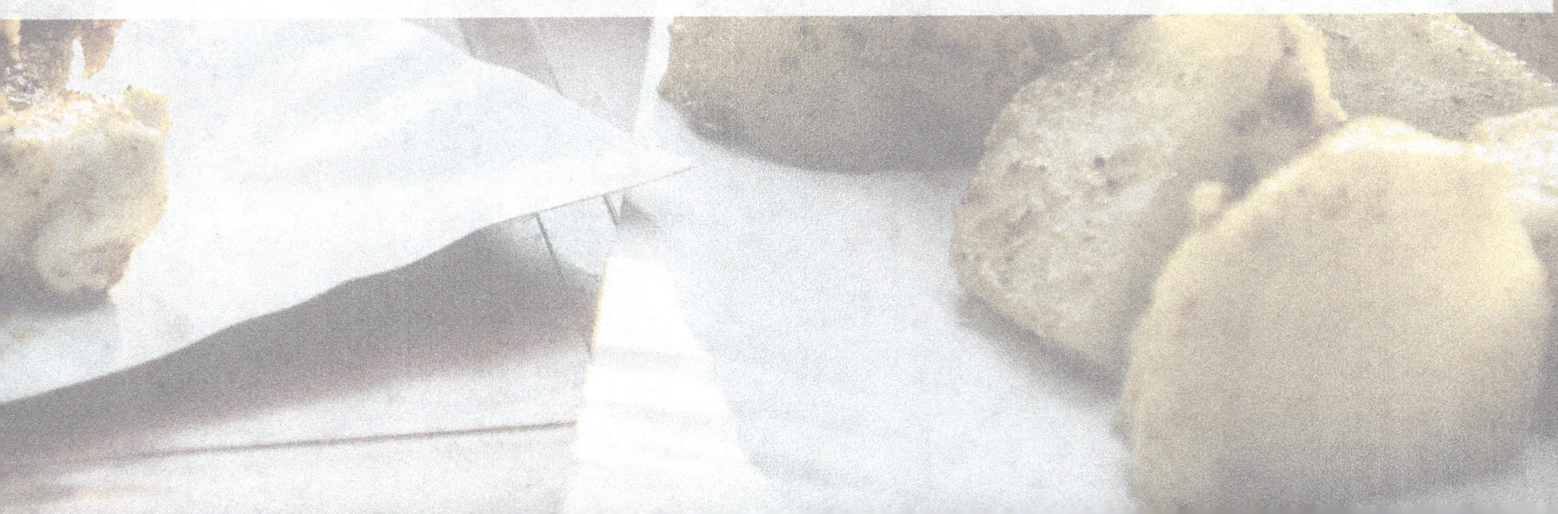